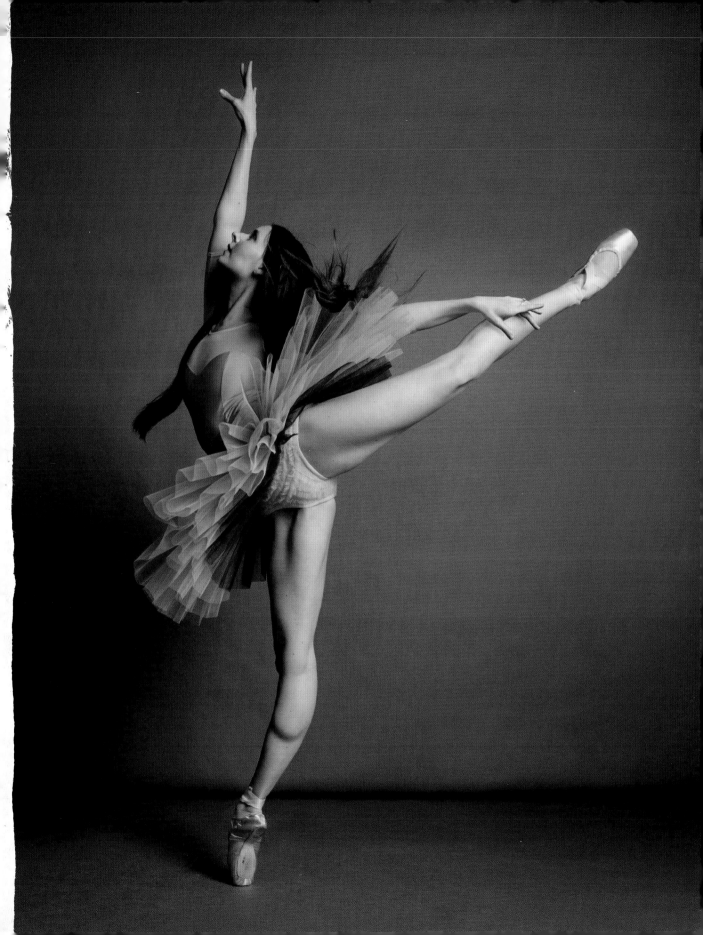

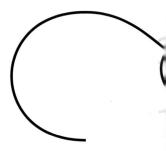

To Lumina and Violette,
may your every dream come true.

And to the many Ballet Beauties
around the world,
may your days be filled with dance!

Ballet for Life

EXERCISES AND INSPIRATION
FROM THE WORLD
OF BALLET BEAUTIFUL

Principal photography by
Inez and Vinoodh

Additional photography by
Chris Colls
Harry Zernike

Mary Helen Bowers

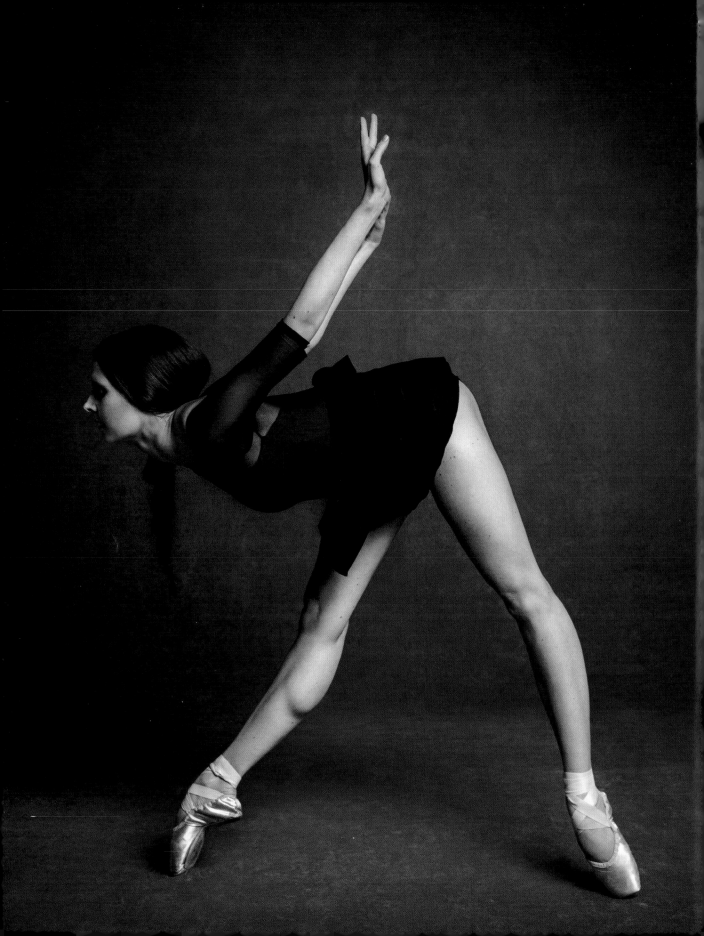

Contents

15 *Foreword*

19 *Introduction*

25 PART ONE: A BALLET BEAUTIFUL BODY

29 *Legs*

47 *Feet*

67 *Center*

85 *Derrière*

105 *Posture*

123 *Flexibility*

145 PART TWO: A BALLET BEAUTIFUL LIFE

149 *Style*

161 *Beauty*

173 *Kitchen*

186 *Glossary*

189 *Acknowledgments*

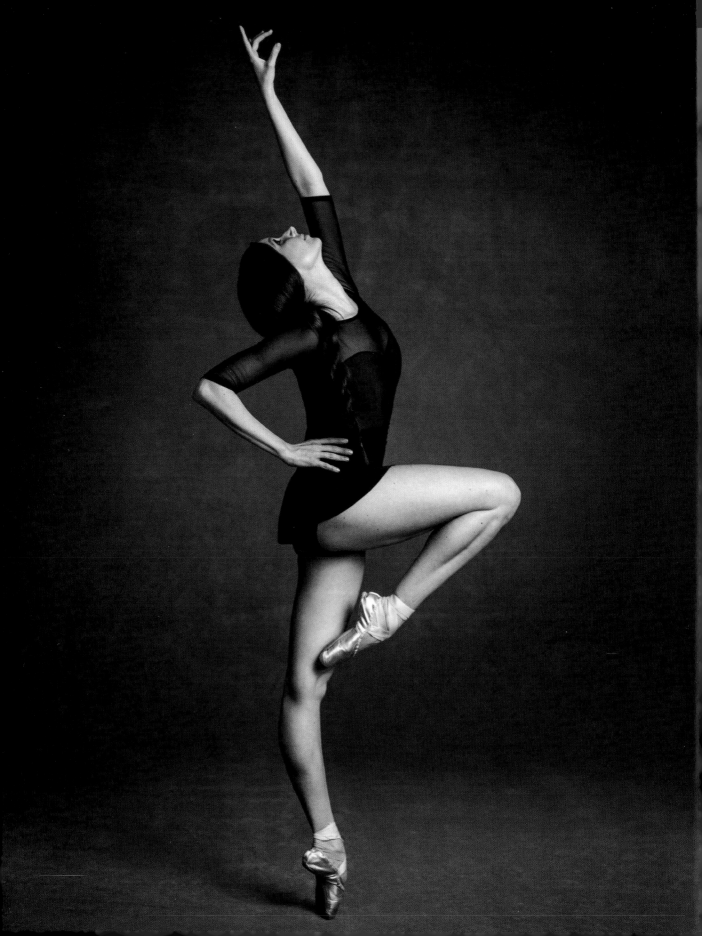

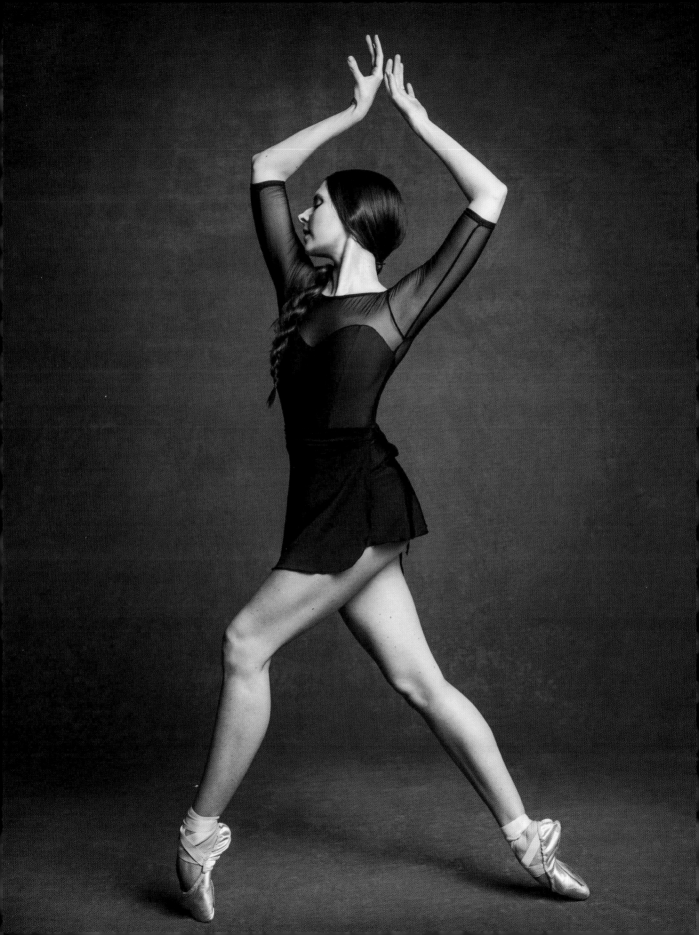

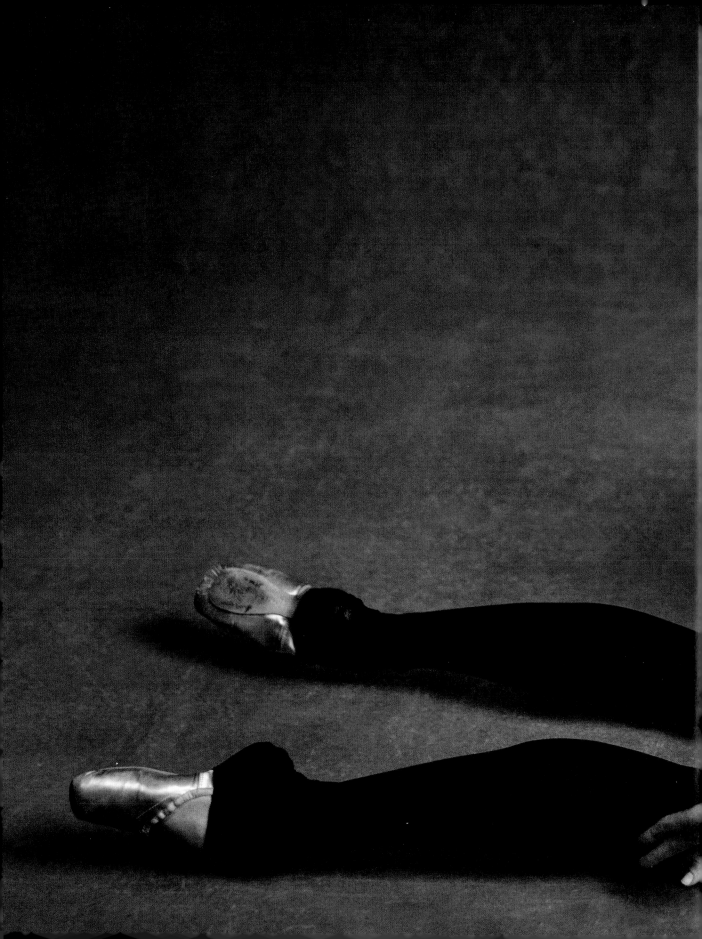

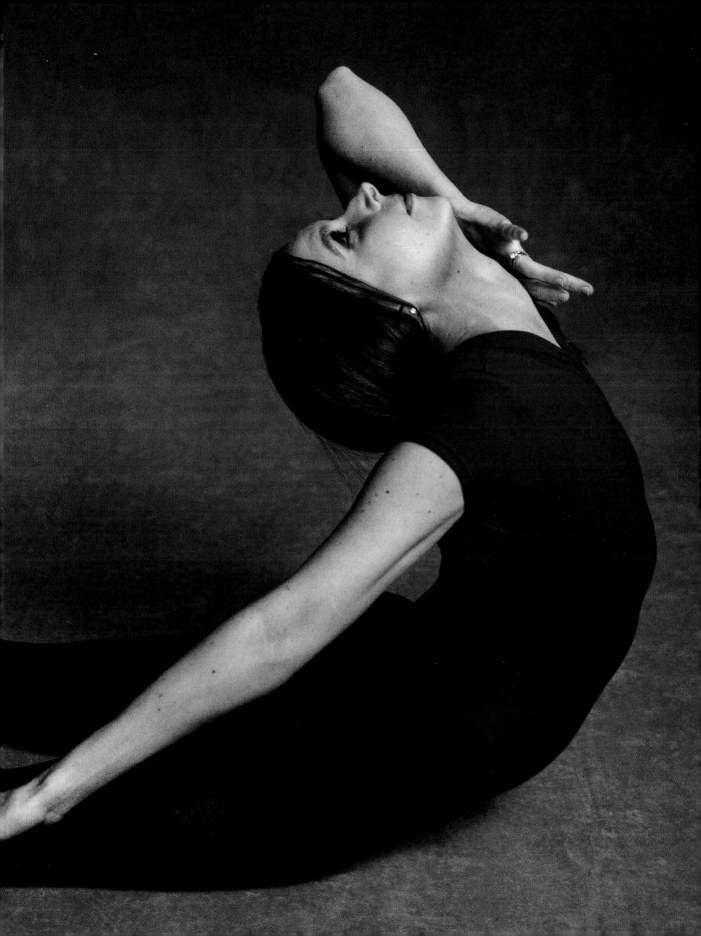

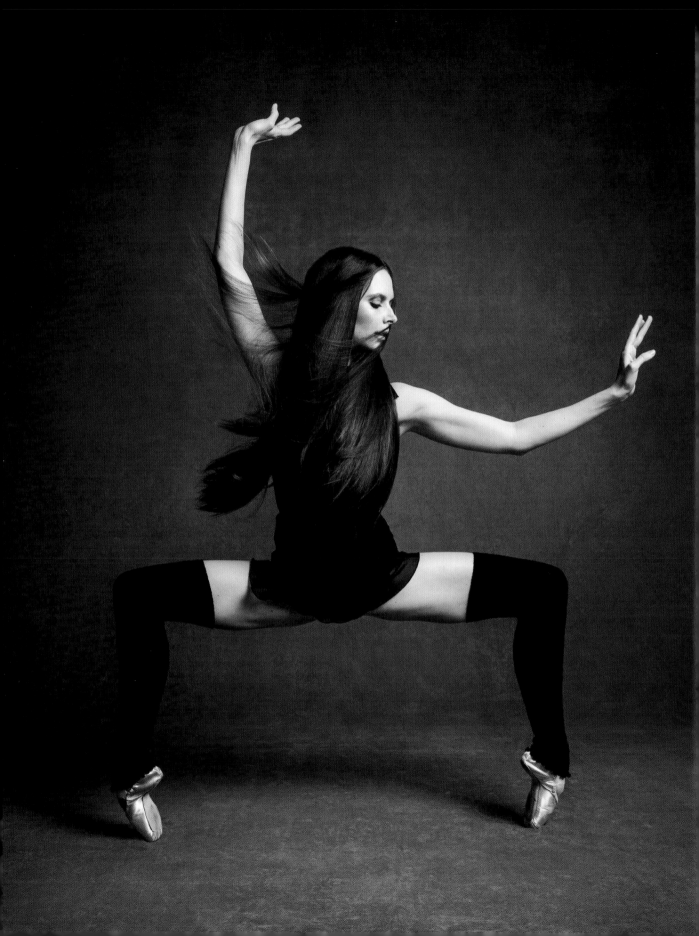

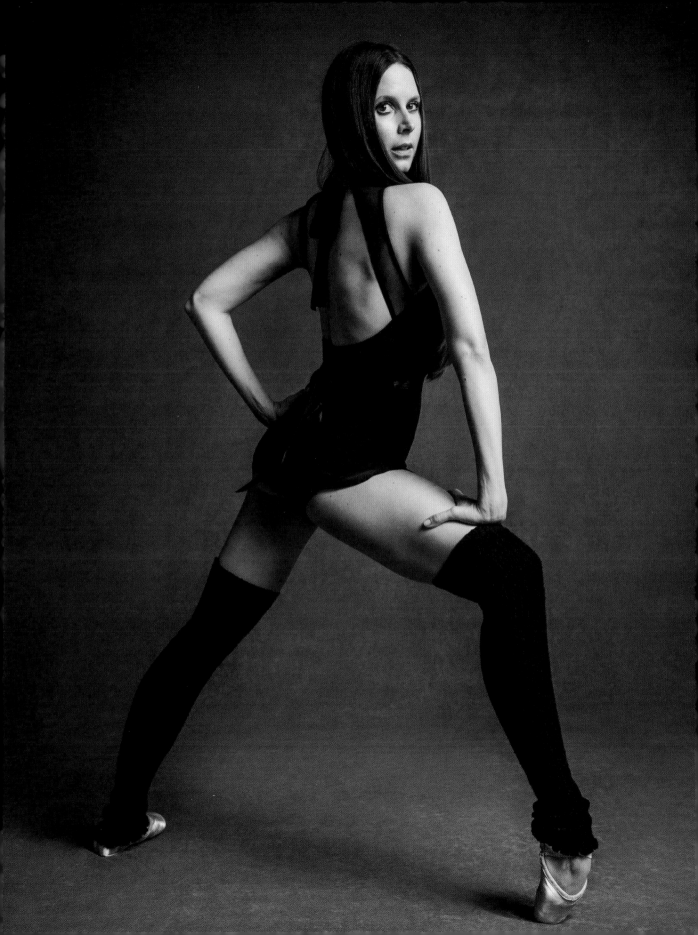

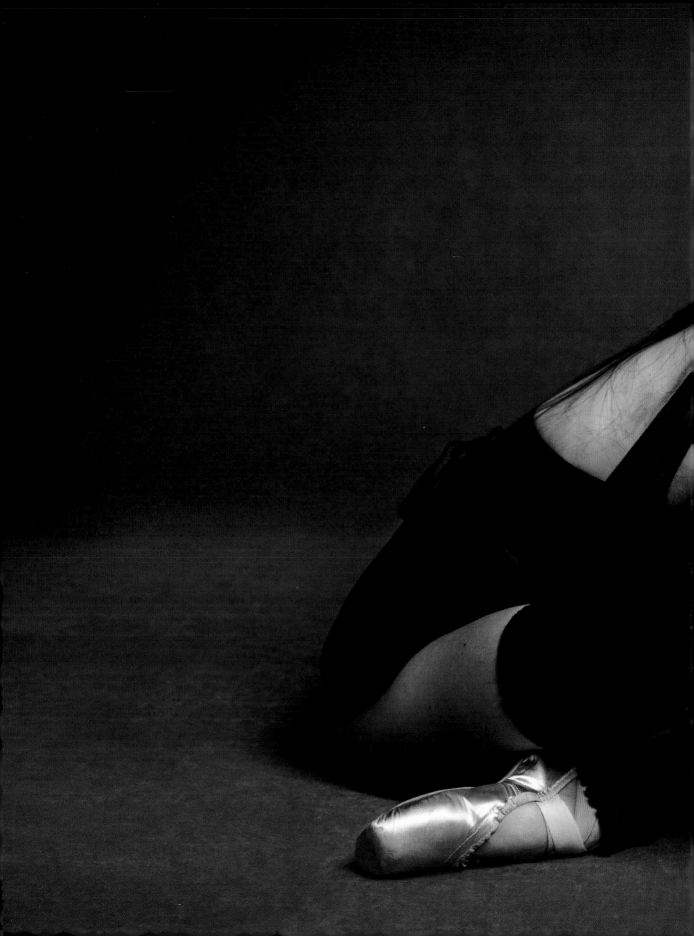

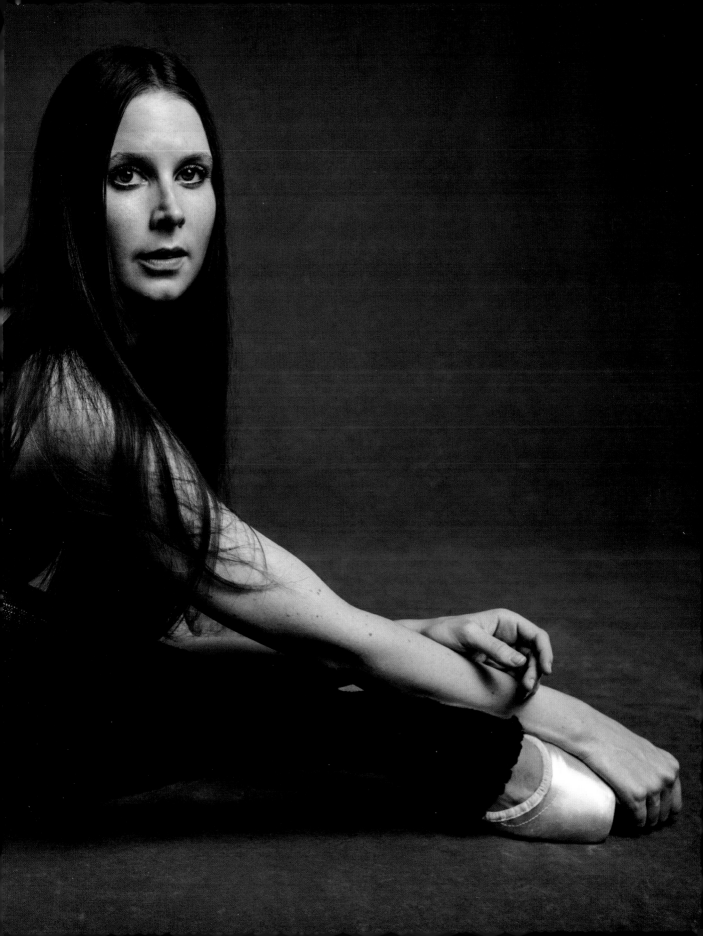

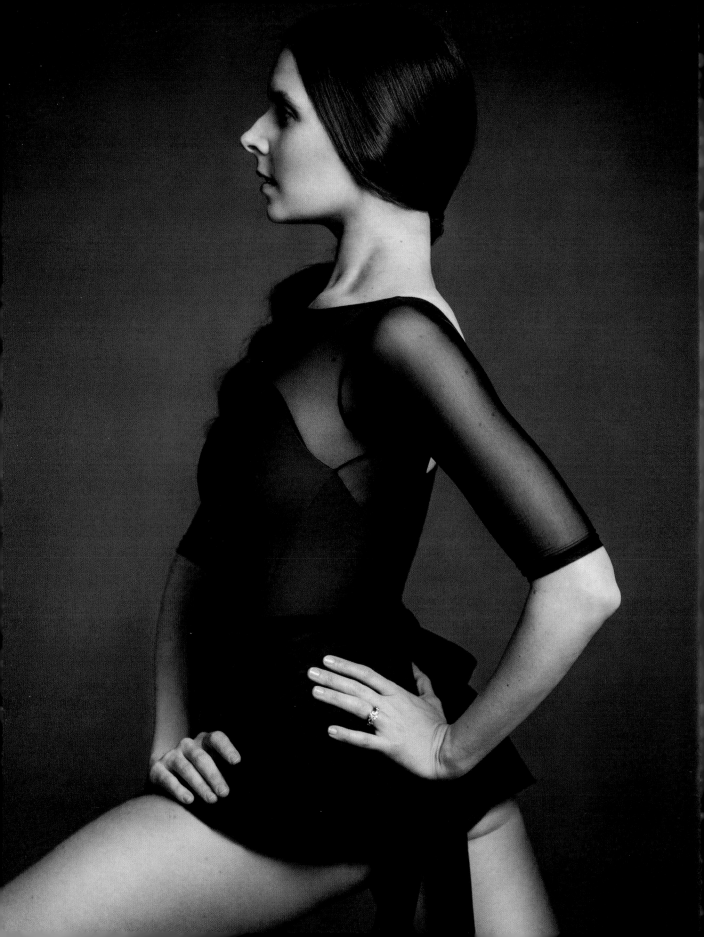

Foreword

*T*he first time I saw Mary Helen was when she walked into my gym for our initial workout. I'd seen her on Instagram but in person she blew me away with her grace and poise. I had reached out to her to train me shortly after my daughter Dixie was born in order to get back in shape for a Victoria's Secret fashion show. The baby was only two months old and I had two months to get runway ready.

Mary Helen told me, "No problem." Then she slipped on her ballet slippers and we started the workout. I'll never forget that first Ballet Beautiful workout—how incredibly hard it was and how sore my muscles felt the next day. I could feel my body changing. Day by day, week by week, we kept training, building strength and muscle tone. We used muscles in my inner thighs, butt, and core that I didn't even know I had. I could see my abs forming (the best feeling after having a baby), my legs leaning out, and my muscles gaining overall tone and condition. By the time the show was upon us I had never felt more confident in my body! I was strong and lean but still had my curves. I had done it all while nursing my young daughter and nourishing my body with the healthiest foods I could find. The moment I stepped back onstage after giving birth I felt so proud. All the hard work had paid off! I could not have done it without Mary Helen and her positive attitude and outlook.

Four years later, we still train almost every day. Since then Mary Helen has had two beautiful baby girls. While she was pregnant she inspired me in a whole new way, continuing to work and train through both pregnancies, always with a smile on her face and a positive attitude. The workouts are still as hard as that first day, but as moms, we speed through each one talking about our babies—their sleeping habits, favorite foods, even the best school options! Mary Helen is my trainer, best friend, and confidante, and an overall inspiration.

I am definitely not a ballerina but I love the way that Mary Helen and Ballet Beautiful have made dance a part of my everyday life. Our workouts opened up the world of ballet to me, inspiring my wardrobe, exercising, and how I move through my day. Whether I am practicing my *pliés*, working on my "Swan Arms," or even just slipping on my ballet shoes and leotard for a workout, the grace inherent in Ballet Beautiful always leaves me uplifted and inspired.

Thank you, Mary Helen. Love you,

Lily

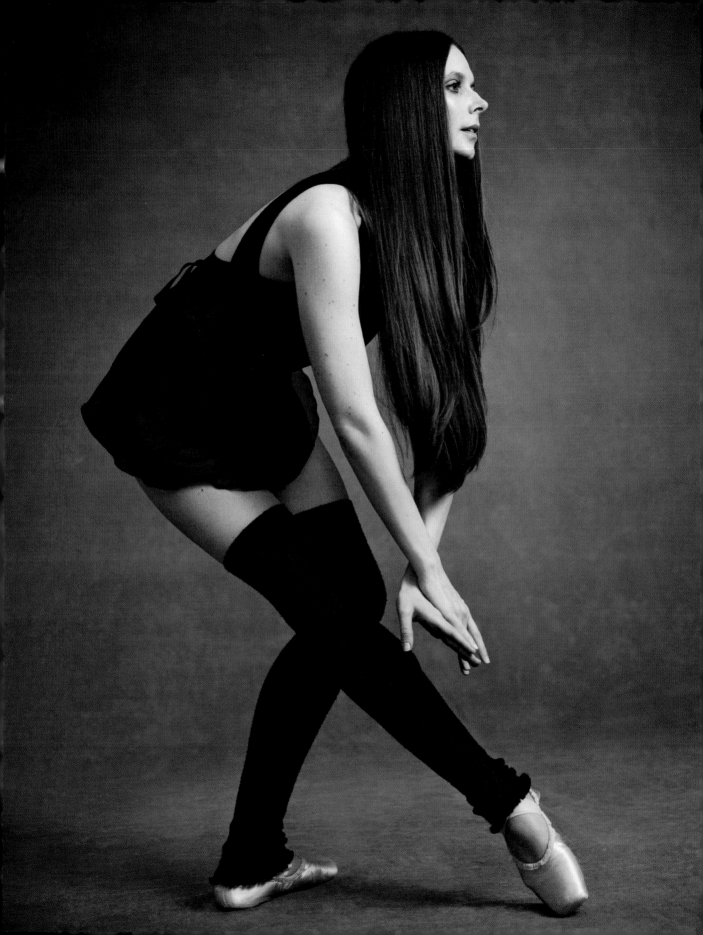

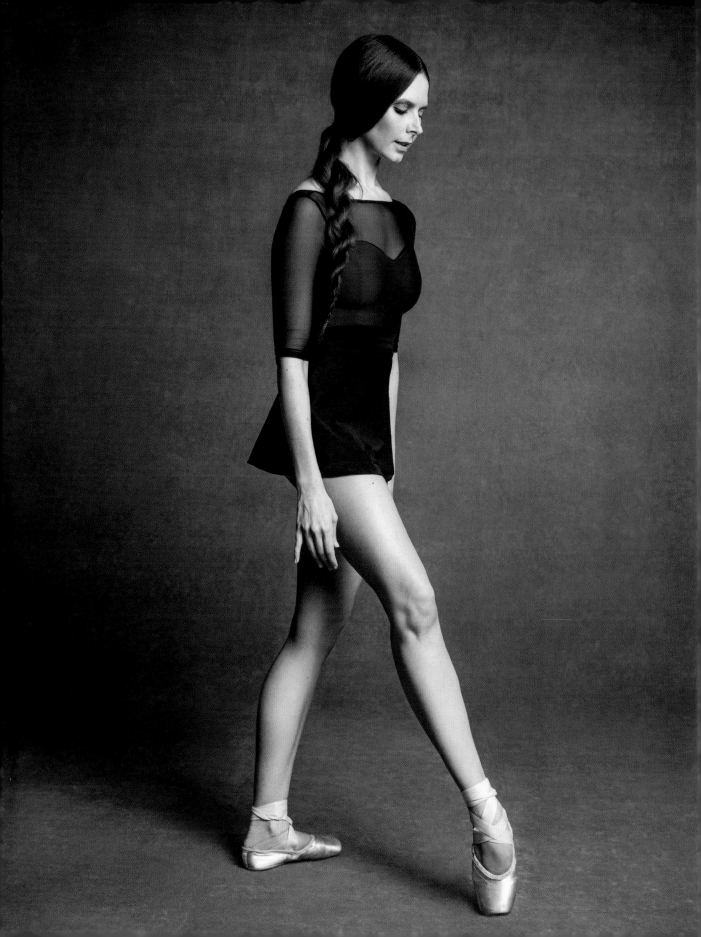

Introduction

Most nights I dream that I am dancing. Sometimes I am in class working furiously on my technique, searching for that perfect extension or grand jeté. *In some dreams I am backstage, racing against the ringing of the theater's warning bells to finish putting on my eyeliner and pin up my hair and headpiece before the curtain rises. But more often than not, I dream that I am onstage under the brilliance of the lights, my feet* en pointe *and my body seemingly weightless. Floating through space, I am entwined with the music.*

Ballet is in many ways my first true love. Deeply woven into the fabric of my body and my life, my love for dance is an inseparable part of me. Like any classic love story, ballet has brought me incredible joy, but also pain across the years, with cherished dreams crushed and made along the way.

I've been dancing since I was a child. Long before I began to study ballet I was dancing through our suburban neighborhood, spinning across the kitchen floor at home and waltzing my way down the supermarket aisles. And yet I cannot explain exactly what first drew me to ballet or why I have always loved it with such intensity. There are no dancers or professional artists in my family. My parents are about as far from stage parents as two could be. I grew up in a happy home, a two-story brick house centered on a leafy cul-de-sac in Charlotte, North Carolina, with two older brothers and both parents working full-time.

While I have always loved to dance, it wasn't until the summer that I was seven years old that I began to think about enrolling in ballet. My friends and I were in the midst of a highly competitive handstand contest at our neighborhood pool. These same friends were ballet obsessed and insisted on including dance in the contest. I won the toe-pointing portion for best handstand, yet had never formally studied ballet. Even though my friends and I were just a group of kids being silly in the pool, I loved the feeling of pointing my feet with everything I had, and extending my legs as long and high as I could through the water. Suddenly I was connecting with my body in this incredible new way, and together we were speaking an exotic foreign language. In that moment I realized that somehow, even while upside down in a swimming pool, I stood out from the crowd. Once home, I pleaded with my mom to let me take ballet classes. I was enrolled by the time fall began.

Like many young girls, I started with one introductory-level class a week but before long I was head over heels in love with my training, spending five or six days a week in the ballet studio, becoming more serious and dedicated with each passing year. By the time I was a preteen, all my free time was spent at ballet. While my friends entering middle school were obsessed with boys, sports, and popularity, my sights were set on dancing with a professional ballet company in New York City. To my family and friends in Charlotte this must have seemed like a far-flung dream. But I have never been too concerned about doing the conventional thing. I simply wanted to dance, even if doing so would mean leaving home and everything familiar to me.

When I received an offer to study as a full-scholarship student at the School of American Ballet in New York City, I never once questioned if it was the right path for me.

I was fifteen and entering my sophomore year of high school. The answer was a booming *"yes."* Of course I would be there! Convincing my parents to allow me to move to New York City as a high school sophomore took a bit more work, but my parents are nothing if not supportive of my dreams. They did everything they could to make it happen, applying my college funds toward the fees for my dormitory and the expensive private school that would allow me to study dance as a pre-professional and finish high school at the same time. From that point on I never looked back.

As a young dancer I simply danced. I did not worry about how my body functioned or why. I was a true "ballet nerd" who had never had a sip of alcohol, gone on a date, or missed a curfew. I was interested in one thing only: ballet. I spent just a little over a year training at the School of American Ballet before being invited to join New York City Ballet's company for the winter season at age sixteen. Dancing with New York City Ballet was my ultimate dream. I was honored and elated to be performing with the world-famous company for the first time, as a Snowflake from *The Nutcracker* in the opening-night gala in Lincoln Center. Even now I smile when I remember the incredible excitement I felt the first time I stepped onstage at Lincoln Center. It was not, however, until my first stage rehearsal that I began to comprehend the incredible athleticism of professional ballet dancers.

Thinking back, I can almost feel the sharpness of the cold air my first time onstage. The heavy crimson curtain was open, with cool air blowing in from the front of the house and nervous energy in the air. My muscles were still warm from company class in the main hall upstairs at what was then called the New York State Theatre (currently the Koch Theatre) that morning, making the contrast more extreme. The stage itself was so much larger than I had imagined. It was an orchestra rehearsal with the company director, Peter Martins, and the first time we would run the piece all the way through. In the handful of rehearsals that I had had with the company up to this point, we would often stop (and briefly rest) for corrections, to adjust the tempo with the pianist, or to make other spacing or technical changes. I was only a teenager, just starting my junior year in high school. I never could have conceived of what was physically in store for me. As a taller dancer I was cast in the "tall girls" section of the Snowflakes, whose dance at the end of Act I is known for being "puffy," a dance term for a highly aerobic piece that leaves you "puffed," or out of breath. By the end of the first run-through I could no longer feel my feet. The veteran dancers were flushed and slightly out of breath, but I was panting and my legs were numb. I thought that I might possibly die right there onstage. Then, after a few quick corrections for the orchestra and dancers, we were asked to repeat it again from the top. I wondered how my feet and legs would get me through not only the rest of that morning rehearsal, but the show that night. I survived those run-throughs but felt fear instead of confidence about my body. In the hours before the show that night I wondered how I would make it through the performance. Was I ready to be out onstage with my idols like Wendy Whelan and Albert Evans? What should I eat to give myself more energy? How could my inexperienced teenage body possibly keep up with the professionals?

When the curtain lifted that evening and I found myself onstage, a true New York City ballerina in Lincoln Center, my anxiety and exhaustion melted with the notes of the music. I felt elated, practically floating across the stage. I vividly remember the utter delight I felt and how intensely beautiful the theater and audience looked. I loved the mystery and intimacy of dancing before the velvety darkness of the audience contrasting with the brilliant stage lights. Performing is almost like dancing with your eyes closed—it's more about the feeling and experience of dance than technique. There's a magical chemistry between you, your fellow dancers, the musicians, and the audience that comes together in an adrenaline-packed rush. As I sailed through the choreography onstage, I learned about the power of adrenaline and the lifesaving lift that it can give a fatigued and, in my case, inexperienced young dancer.

As my career progressed I came into my own as a dancer. I learned how to connect with and push my body onstage as well as how to take care of it when offstage. Those days as a young dancer were the early phases of my beginning to understand my body as a ballerina, an athlete, and a woman. But while I bloomed as an artist I also suffered setbacks, like injuries and weight gain. I started Gyrotonics and swimming, joined a gym, and, for the first time, began working out outside of a dance studio. I learned that in addition to my daily ballet class, rehearsals, and performing, my body needed cross-training and additional strengthening to build stamina and help prevent injury. Finding a ballet-friendly program proved more difficult than I had imagined. Dancing alone was not enough, but I had to be very careful not to overwork my body or build muscles in the wrong places. I tried everything—yoga, kickboxing, Pilates, spinning, even boot-camp classes—always modifying the workouts for my body as a ballerina. The program that I needed didn't exist in any class at the gym and so I began creating a mini workout system for myself to use at home in the mornings or backstage between rehearsals or a show. I took my time developing my routine, noting what worked and what didn't, tweaking and adjusting it along the way. Once I figured out the right formula, I was amazed by how strong and uplifted each workout made me feel. My body felt powerful yet light, and, ultimately, so did my mind. The stage was set for the world that would one day become Ballet Beautiful.

It is not easy to bid a dream farewell, and leaving New York City Ballet was one of the most agonizing decisions of my life. After ten intense years of love and toil, blisters and injuries and total bliss, it was hard for me to imagine that there would be a place for ballet in my life outside of a professional company. But after I retired and enough time had passed to heal my exhausted body and mind, I felt a little bit empty without dance in my life. I fought the feeling at first but there was no denying that my body craved movement, and so did my heart. I returned to my mini workouts, but instead of practicing backstage I found a space for myself in my bedroom or in between classes at the gym at Columbia University, where I was pursuing my Bachelor of Arts.

For the first time in many years I didn't feel any pressure to move or look a certain way, be it in my leotard or a pair of jeans. Exercise became a new and unexpected creative outlet as I experimented with and expanded upon my workouts. I meshed fitness favorites, like lunges and abdominal work, with classical ballet training, always with a dancer's body in mind. My body's response was immediate. I felt strong again, but now with a new confidence. After spending years dancing and training with New York City Ballet for ten to twelve hours a day, I was amazed to see my ballet muscles reemerge as my body tightened and changed shape with only an hour or less of exercise a few days a week.

I never realized how much I had missed ballet until I began reconnecting with it. What started out as simply picking up my workout again began to seep into other parts of my life. First there was the wardrobe. I found myself wearing my ballet clothes again but now with a new purpose outside the ballet studio. I can't say that I missed my pointe shoes (ouch!), but there's no question that I craved the glamour and allure of my daily dose of satin slippers. I began discovering a way to bring ballet back into my life, but this time under my own terms. As I built a new life for myself I came to see that ballet could be a part of my life, without being the only thing in my life. This new perspective was totally unexpected. I realized that it was changing the way I saw not only the world but also the role that ballet had always played for me. Suddenly I began to relax. I began to understand that I am always a dancer, even when I am not onstage. We all are! This thinking was radically different from the all-consuming life of a ballerina that I had previously known. In it I found freedom, happiness, and, most importantly, a life filled with Ballet Beauty—and I wanted to share it with others.

A movement began to grow as I shared my workouts with family and friends and they too experienced changes in their bodies and lives. Friends told friends and before I knew it I was building a business, one client at a time. It was early in this process that I met Natalie Portman and we began training for her role in Darren Aronofsky's *Black Swan*. With my young business and flexible schedule, the timing was perfect for taking on this intense project that demanded Natalie and I travel together across the world, spending five-plus hours a day, six days a week, training and preparing for her transformation into a ballerina on the screen. I could not have asked for a more devoted student. Natalie's incredible work ethic and discipline rival that of any dancer I have ever met.

I was constantly on the go and found that the same was true for my clients. When I wasn't working with Natalie, I was training online with clients back home in New York City or Los Angeles. Working online from an apartment or hotel, I was connecting with clients doing the same—no weights, equipment, or ballet barre required. The process of creating and building the business was a fluid one. I was continually developing and expanding Ballet Beautiful with this busy, modern client in mind. We all had the same goal: to strengthen and transform our bodies with a workout that was inspiring and fun. I intensified and condensed the workouts, focusing on getting the most out of an hour of exercise, regardless of location. From there it was simply a question of how to share Ballet Beautiful with others and build a business with true scale. The learning curve was steep but I was doing what I loved. After so many years of being told how to look and what to do, I relished both the creativity and control that I felt as a businesswoman. I began building a team to help me design and launch our website, produce our first streaming workouts and DVDs, and open our flagship SoHo studio, introducing Ballet Beautiful to the world.

To me ballet is everything that is beautiful, and dancing is an expression of love. The secret to Ballet Beautiful is incorporating the magical elements of ballet into daily life, from how we work out to our daily fashions and style to the way we eat and live. Exercise can be both inspiring and artistic, tapping into dormant "ballet" muscles to awaken and reshape the body as never before. The picture is complete with ballet clothes that add just the right amount of chic to any look, along with the perfectly placed flower, satin slipper, or dash of tulle to bring light and grace to any room.

With Ballet Beautiful I've chosen to focus on my favorite aspects of what it means to be a ballerina: health, beauty, and empowerment. The goal of Ballet Beautiful, and this book, is to share this vision of ballet and to experience it with others.

Welcome to the world of Ballet Beautiful. I hope you will share in the dream!

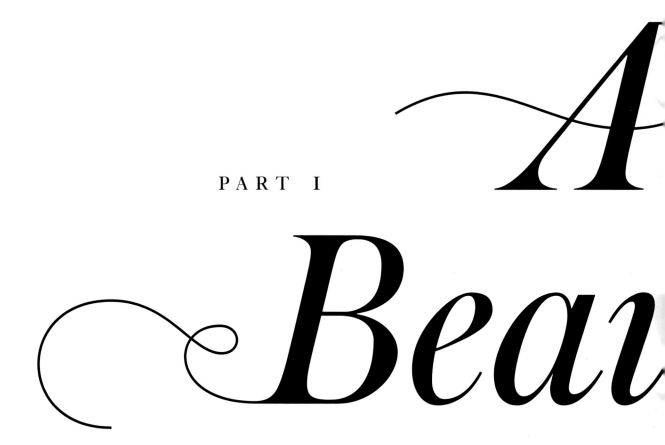

PART I

Ballet

tiful

Body

Ballet dancers are a singular combination of artist and athlete; there is no art form as purely physical as ballet. As a result, the connection between a dancer and her body is a powerful one. Carefully sculpted through countless hours in the studio and years of disciplined training, a dancer's body is her instrument. Lean, taut muscles, incredible flexibility, and regal posture are a dancer's calling card. Each muscle has a purpose; each callus is hard earned.

Ballet speaks to parts of us that are both powerful and delicate. Although classical ballet may appear soft at first glance, it is driven by a potent physical energy. This seeming dichotomy adds to ballet's allure. Ballet captures the very human push and pull between strength and softness in each of us. Dancers know better than anyone that movement has the potential to become so much more than just physical activity.

I have always loved dancing and being active, but I never felt inspired at the gym. In fact, physical education was my least favorite subject in school. In middle school I was happy to work on my splits and practice *tendus* and *port de bras* on the balance beam during gymnastics. At the same time, I dreaded almost everything else about gym class. When I became more serious about my ballet training, I refused to kick the ball during soccer drills for fear that I might twist or injure my ankle. My gym teacher saw a stubborn teenager, not a budding ballerina protecting her legs and feet. I may have only been thirteen, but I knew that ballet and soccer did not mix. But ballet was the center of my life. I would not put it at risk for something meaningless to me. I did not relent, enlisting my mom to help me petition for a dismissal from soccer that semester. Less than two years later, I was training and dancing in New York City.

As a young ballerina I was too swept up in my love of dance to appreciate the complex relationship between my body and my art. I knew of course that I needed to eat well and get plenty of rest to feel my best, but it was not until I experienced an injury in my early years with New York City Ballet that I began to understand the fragility of a career built around my body. For a dancer, being injured is a terrifying and humbling experience. Without my body I could not express my art, and without ballet I felt disconnected and lost. I wanted to be onstage dancing, not injured on the sidelines. Developing a way to better care for my body as a ballerina was an important part of my process of healing. It also played a pivotal role in the creation of Ballet Beautiful.

While that early injury was a difficult time in my professional career, it was also an opportunity to learn. Though I was dancing professionally for close to a dozen hours a day, I came to see that cross-training was an essential part of taking care of my body as a ballerina. In order to be my strongest, my body needed to be challenged and moved outside of the dance studio. The trick was finding a ballet-friendly form of exercise to complement and support my dancing without over-taxing my joints or bulking my muscles. It was at this time that I joined a gym and began experimenting with other forms of exercise. A tailor-made class for professional ballerinas did not exist, so I sampled what was available, modifying each workout for my body as a dancer.

Before creating Ballet Beautiful, I spent what must have been hundreds of hours on cardio machines. I flirted with spinning, kickboxing, and boot-camp-style workouts. I even tried yoga and Pilates. As a dancer, I was always frustrated by the results from other methods, never happy with how the workouts made me look or feel. I found the energy behind many of these programs to be aggressive. The workouts themselves were too harsh and worked the wrong muscles for a ballerina. Even the accompanying music was too loud. During this time, I was careful to avoid lifting any weights over five pounds in order to keep my upper body toned but lean. I eschewed using machines and any exercise that targeted the quads to prevent overbuilding my thighs. Extra stretching kept my muscles loose and long. I changed exercises as needed in an effort not to over-train or bulk my legs or upper body, or drastically alter my dancer's form. Slowly, I began creating my own ballet-focused workout to strengthen and tone.

What I learned along the way is that much like dancing, exercise can be both inspiring and artistic. A great workout should empower you to look and feel your best, to train harder and stretch farther every day. It shouldn't be a punishment, and it should never feel like a chore. Exercise does not have to involve pounding your body to painful limits, or getting screamed at or shamed at the gym. When mixed with ballet, exercise can express the incredible power and grace inherent in each of us.

I created Ballet Beautiful as a way to strengthen the body and incorporate my favorite aspects of ballet into a workout for anyone. The goal of Ballet Beautiful is to share this ballet-inspired world and help others to live a healthy, active, and dance-filled life.

The Ballet Beautiful approach to training is twofold. First: target the muscles that ballerinas use in everyday training. Ballet-inspired legwork focuses on toning and strengthening the inner thighs and backs of the legs rather than the quadriceps muscles at the front of the thighs, which are quick to thicken and overdevelop. Upper-body exercises are performed from an open, upright position to build beautiful posture and tone without bulking the arms. Pulling the abdominal muscles in tightly throughout each movement strengthens and engages the center without overdeveloping the abdominals. Second: use a ballet-based approach to moving the body. Where most fitness workouts focus on contracting muscles (think squats, crunches, curls, and even the cobra and warrior positions in yoga), ballet centers around *extending* the body through space, stretching long through the arms and legs, from the fingertips to toes. Muscles are strengthened and lengthened, molding a powerful, ballet-specific physique.

In the pages that follow, you'll find explanations of ballet principles and fitness tips that you can use in your own workout to help you train like a ballerina.

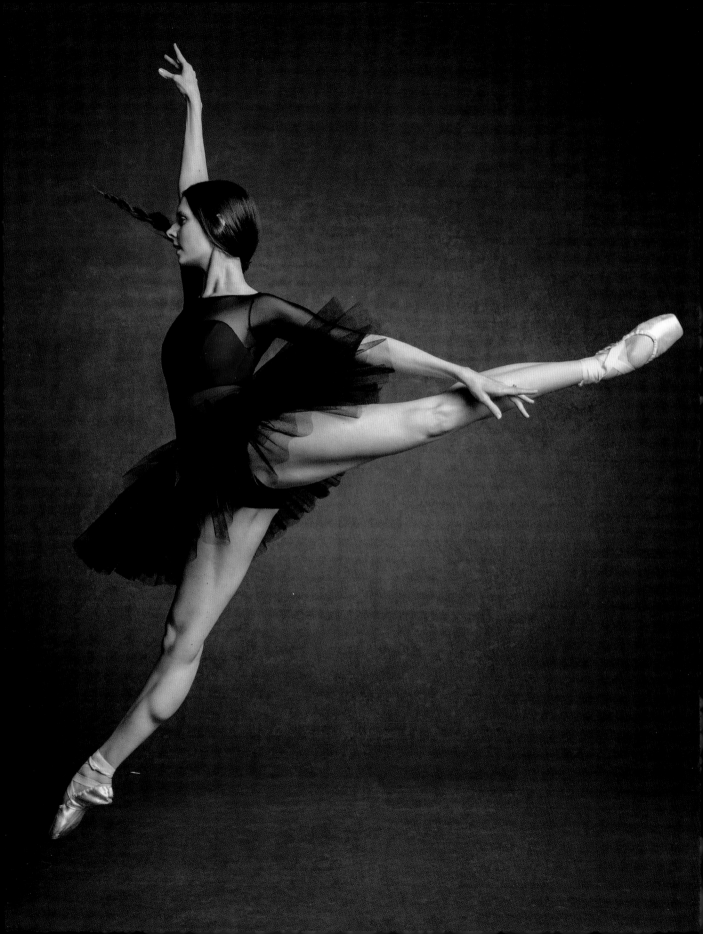

1.1

Legs

*B*eautifully toned, dynamic legs are a dancer's trademark. *Expertly sculpted from a seemingly endless series of* pliés, tendus, *and* arabesques, *legs are also the foundation of a dancer's body and form.*

Nowhere is this more obvious than in George Balanchine's stark "leotard ballets." With dancers costumed in only a practice leotard and tights, save a small belt or skirt, these neoclassical ballets put the body on full display, highlighting the beauty of a dancer's legs and form. Ever since I was a little girl, I had admired these ballets, sitting in the audience or from photographs and videos, but when I began dancing in them, I felt incredibly exposed—and free. The sensation of being onstage with my legs clad only in a pair of pink or white tights was a new one: without the pouf of a tutu or the cover of a costume I felt more connected with my body, the music, and the movement. Of all the leotard ballets in New York City Ballet's repertoire, *The Four Temperaments* was one of my favorites to perform. I loved the feeling of extending all the way through my legs, brushing and kicking with everything I had in the *piqué en arabesque* section from "Phlegmatic" (in the most tranquil way possible, of course).

Imagine a dancer in motion onstage—toes pointed, legs and arms stretched and elongated, every muscle and tendon flexing, lifting, and extending her body through space. This focus on the extension of the legs is a central principle of both classical ballet and Ballet Beautiful training. Working the muscles incredibly hard while stretching them "long" builds muscle that is powerful and lean. From the typical fitness workout perspective, the stretching of the knees that is fundamental in ballet can feel incredibly foreign. Many of us are taught to keep some slack in the knees when working out or lifting weights, but with ballet the opposite is true. Ballet training engages and lifts the knees to stretch and elongate the legs.

Another important difference when contrasting ballet to fitness, or even other genres of dance, is the element of turnout. In ballet, the legs are generally turned out or opened from the hips, actively engaging the inner thighs. Working in this turned-out position adds strength and tone to the inside and backs of the legs without overworking the quadriceps muscles. Ballerinas are famously fussy about their legs and fearful of overworking or bulking the thighs. The quadricepses, some of the largest muscles on the legs and which are quick to bulk and overbuild, are engaged through a series of *pliés* (bends) and extensions (stretches) in this turned-out position, which serves to further strengthen and slim. Outer thigh exercises tighten and tone the sides of the thighs and hips and add extra length to the line of the legs.

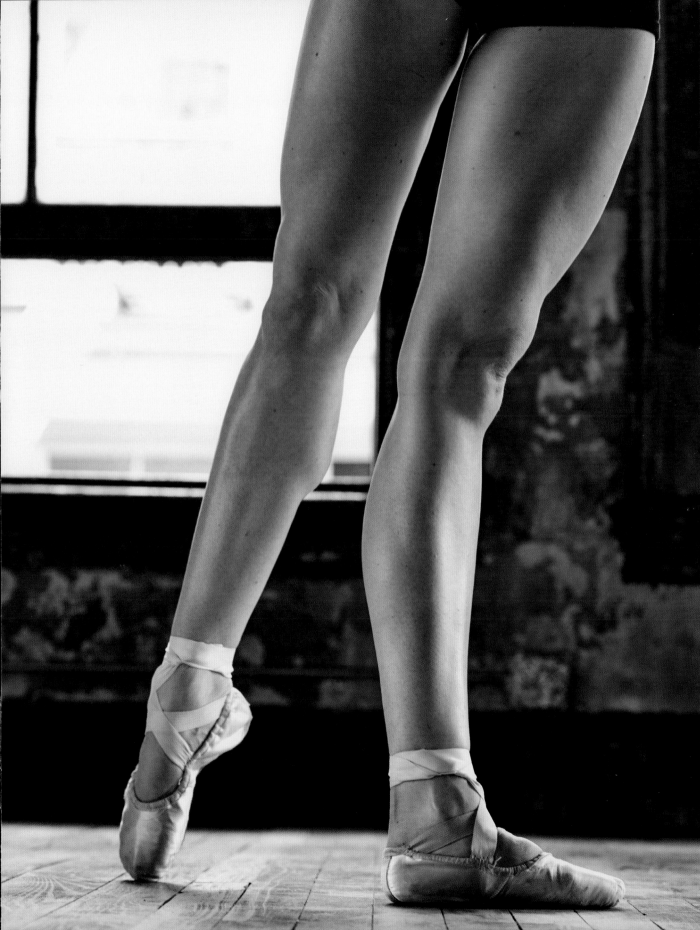

[PREVIOUS PAGE] *Tendu à terre.* A *tendu* is one of the most basic warm-up steps in ballet, typically performed at the barre to the front (*devant*), side (*à la seconde*), and back (*derrière*). *Tendu* means "stretched," and terre means "ground," so *tendu à terre* means "stretched on the ground." This fundamental movement is a simple brushing of the working leg with a pointed toe along the floor, culminating in a stretching of both knees with the working toe remaining on the floor.

Dance Principle
Lift and extend long through both the standing and working legs, stretching from the toes to the hips.

Fitness Tip
Make *tendus* part of your next workout: begin with the heels together in first position. Stretch one leg back into an *arabesque*, pulling in through the core while stretching both legs long. Then close the foot back into first position. Repeat for two sets of eight, and then change sides.

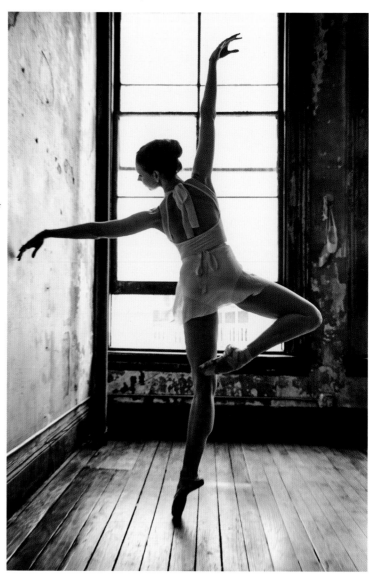

[THIS PAGE + OPPOSITE] A simple *passé en pointe* features both the bend and the stretch that define a dancer's legs. In a *passé* (which means "passed"), the working leg bends and passes along the standing leg, toe to knee, moving into a ninety-degree angle while keeping the working toe against a straight standing knee. A lunge in *à la seconde* with *port de bras* tones and strengthens the inner thighs and waist.

Dance Principle
Keep the toe of the working leg connected to the standing knee *en passé* while opening the working knee from the hip.

Fitness Tip
Incorporate a *piqué passé* in your next workout with this simple lunge series: step onto a straight leg, bending the working knee into *passé*, placing the working toe by the standing knee. Bring the working leg down into a side lunge while bending the arm up and over, away from the working leg (opposite). Open the top arm as you extend the standing leg and step back up into a *passé*. Repeat for two sets of eight, and then change sides.

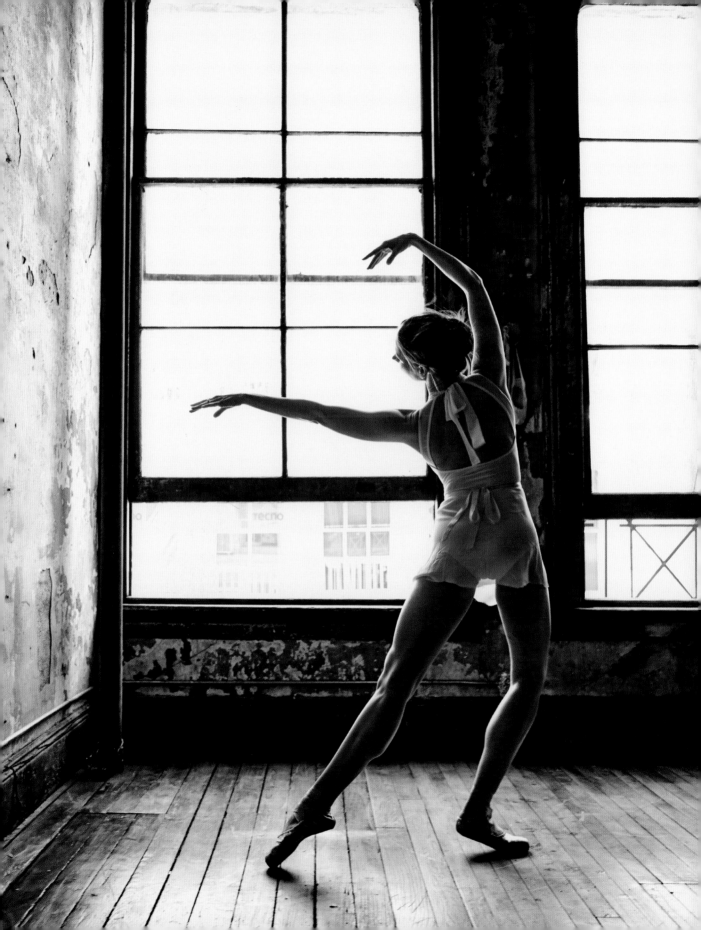

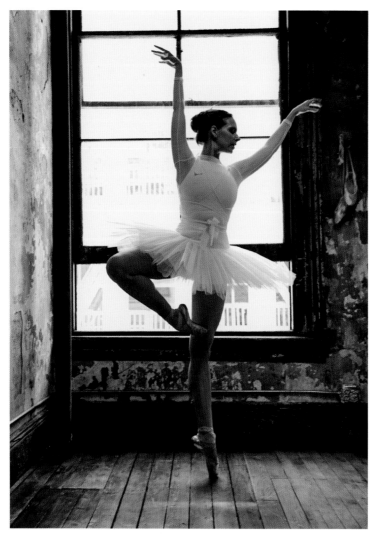

[THIS PAGE] *Plié passé en pointe.*
[OPPOSITE] *Plié tendu* with *cambré en avant.*

[THIS PAGE]
Dance Principle
Lift up and open through the standing and working legs and hips to help with balance on a *plié passé* or *pirouette.*

Pro Tip
Pull in tight through the abdominals and engage the muscles in the back and thighs to control the movement from a lifted *passé en pointe* to a deep forward bend.

Fitness Tip
The greater the range of motion between movements, the more challenging (and cardiovascular) the steps become. Stretch the standing knee and lift the working toe and knee into a *passé.* Lift up and over with arms and the upper body as you melt the standing knee into a *plié* while crossing the wrists and reaching the hands towards the toes. Pull in with the abs and lift the upper body and legs back up and into a *passé* again. Repeat four to eight times, and change sides.

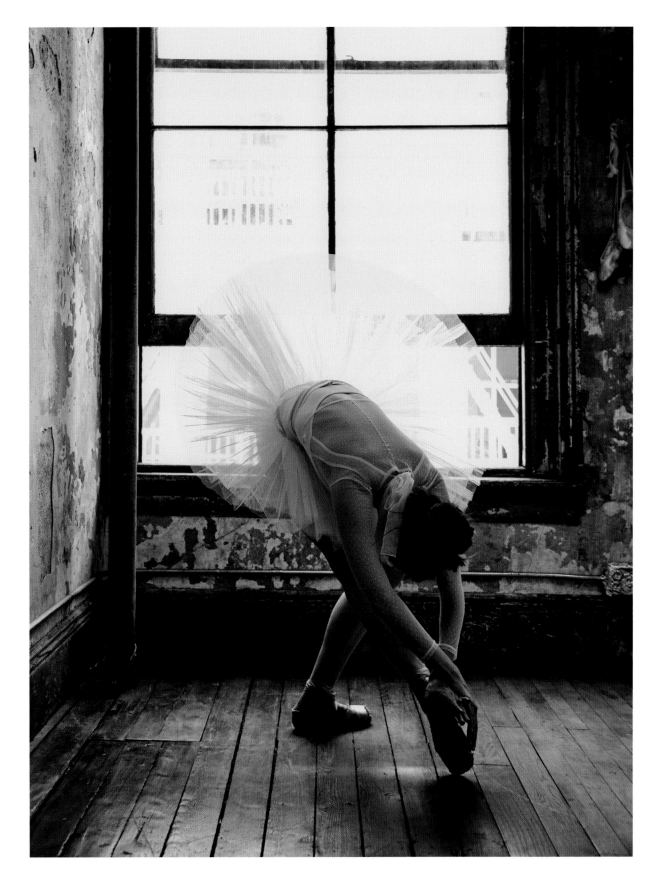

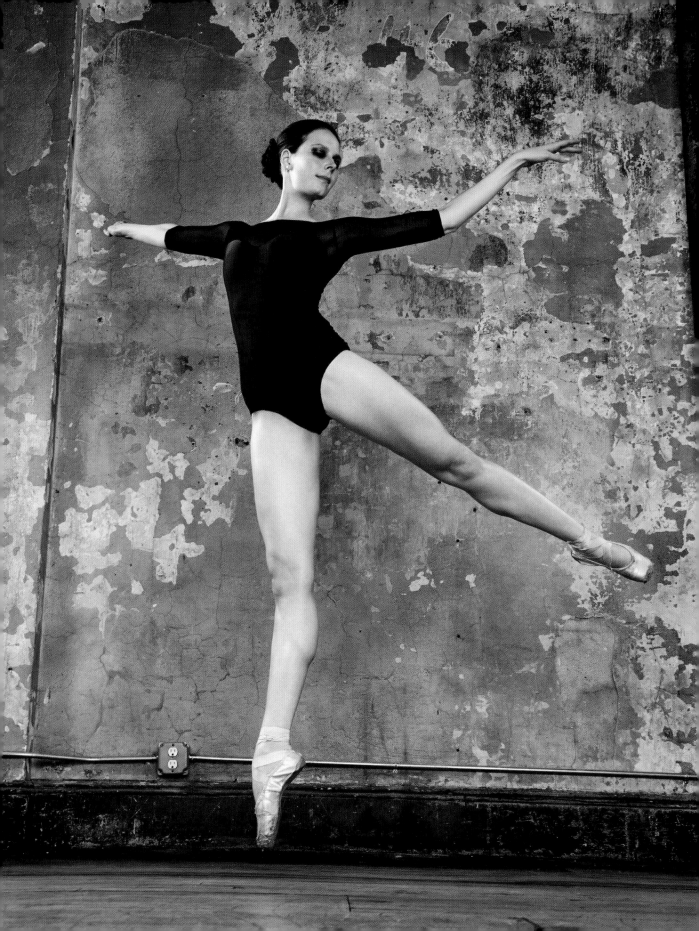

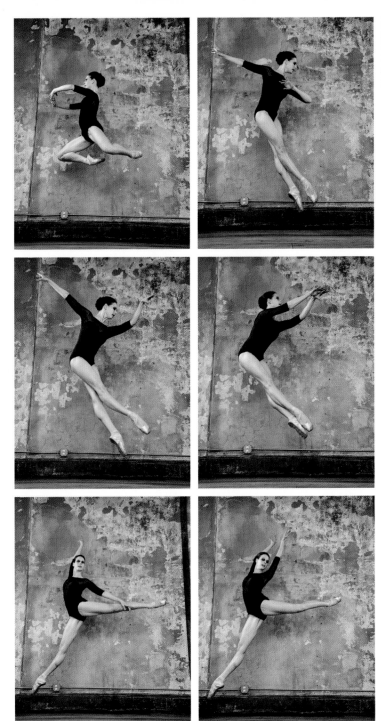

[THIS PAGE + OPPOSITE] Explosive power is required of a dancer's legs when jumping. *Attitude* leaps (this page, top), *assemblé*s (this page, middle), and *sissonne*s (this page, bottom) capture the power of a dancer's legs.

[OPPOSITE] *Sauté arabesque. Sauté*s, meaning "jumps," make for terrific cardio, on or off stage.

Dance Principle
For extra height envision a split second when you "hang" in the air at the top of each jump, freezing the form.

Fitness Tip
Incorporate *sissonne*s into your next workout for serious heart-pounding toning! Begin with the feet together on the floor in a relaxed third position (with the front heel touching the back toe, with the toes slightly open from the hips). Lift the back leg off the floor into *arabesque* while jumping in the air, stretching both knees long and extending the arms out to the side into second position. Repeat four to eight times and change legs.

[FOLLOWING PAGES, FROM LEFT] *Sissonne* in fourth position. *Sissonne arabesque.*

Dance Principle
For your most powerful jumps, place the tension in the legs and core rather than the upper body. Keep the arms and neck relaxed while pushing away from the floor with the legs and toes.

Pro Tip
Picture your full range of motion before taking off. Imagine a photograph being snapped at the top of your jump, capturing your ideal positioning of arms and legs.

37

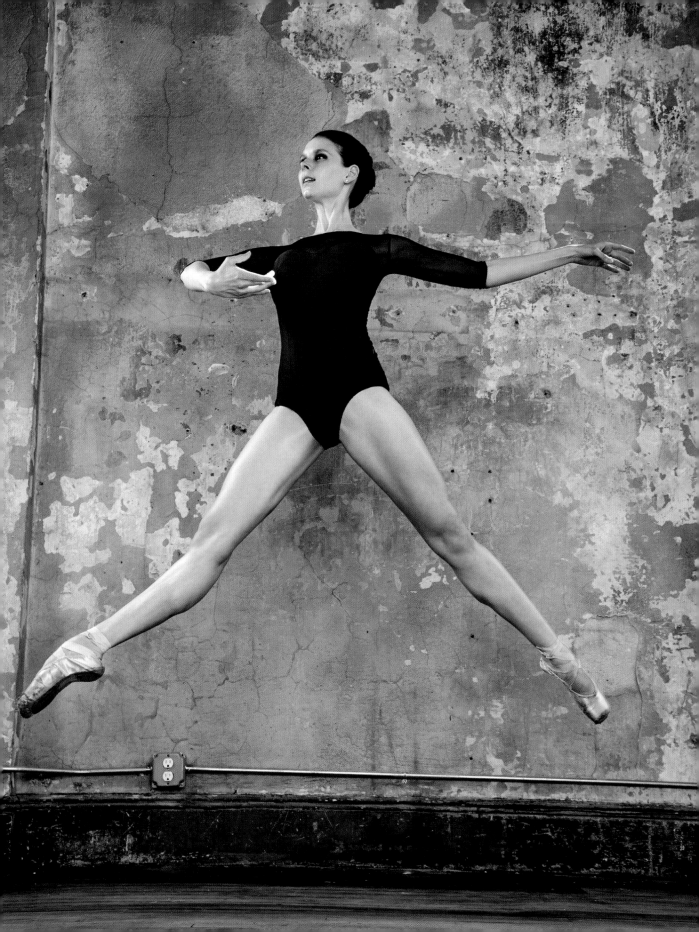

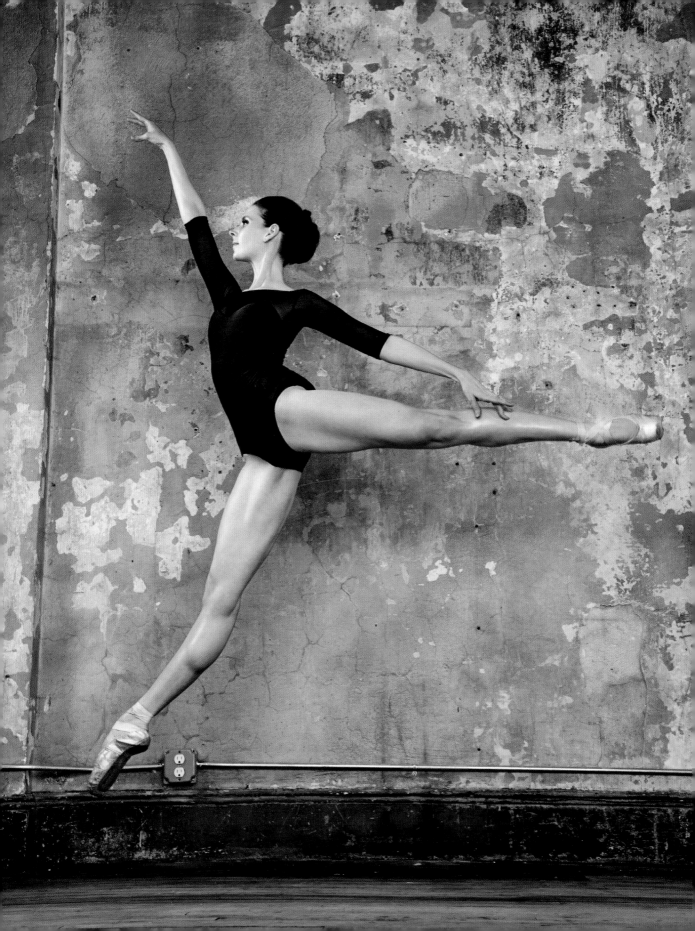

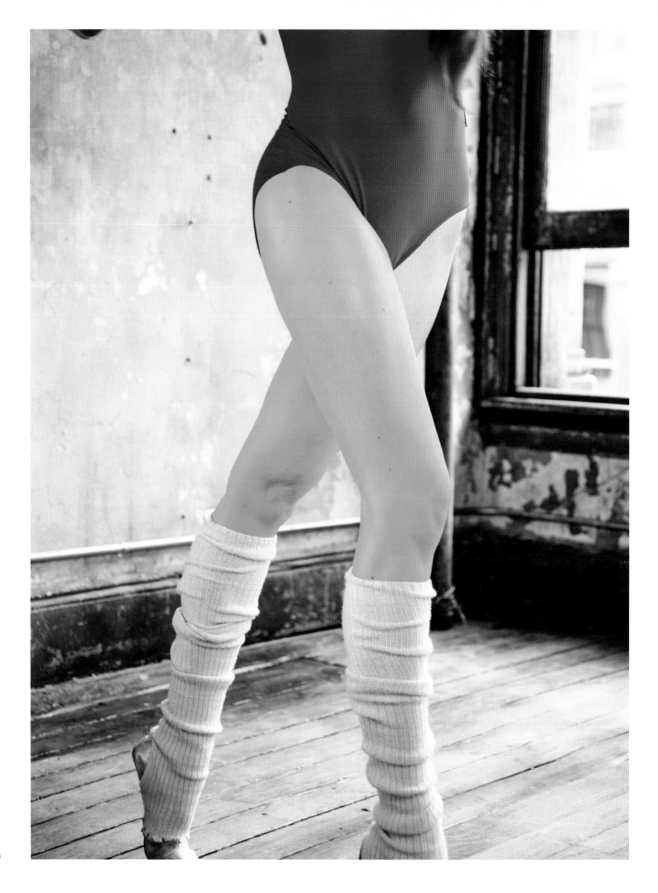

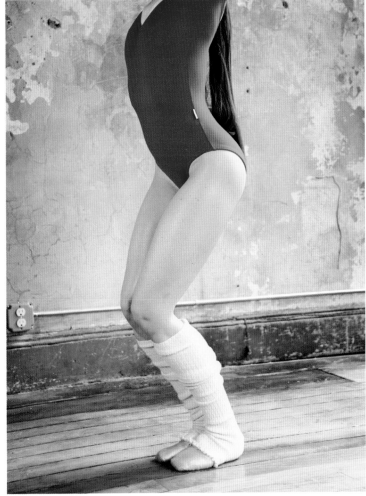

[OPPOSITE] A *tendu* back in parallel lengthens and tones the legs. [THIS PAGE] A simple *plié* in sixth position tones the thighs.

[THIS PAGE]
Dance Principle
Basic movements like a *plié* in sixth position provide the perfect opportunity to catch your breath between steps.

Fitness Tip
Holding a *plié* provides a serious ballet burn! Bring the toes and heels together, pull in tight with the abs, and bend both knees. Hold three to four sets of eight. Add an extra layer of challenge by moving into a *tendu arabesque* on *demi-pointe*. Lift up onto a *demi-pointe* and extend one leg straight back into an *arabesque* to engage and challenge the calves, center, and butt. Repeat for two sets of eight, and then change sides.

[FOLLOWING PAGES] *Passé*, on the floor.

Fitness Tip
Floor and mat work is a terrific way to strengthen and engage your ballet muscles. Lie on one side, and stretch the bottom leg long while bending the top knee into a *passé*. Pull in tight with the abdominals to balance as you lower the working leg from a *passé* to a straight knee in first position. Lift the top knee into *passé* again. Repeat four times and change sides.

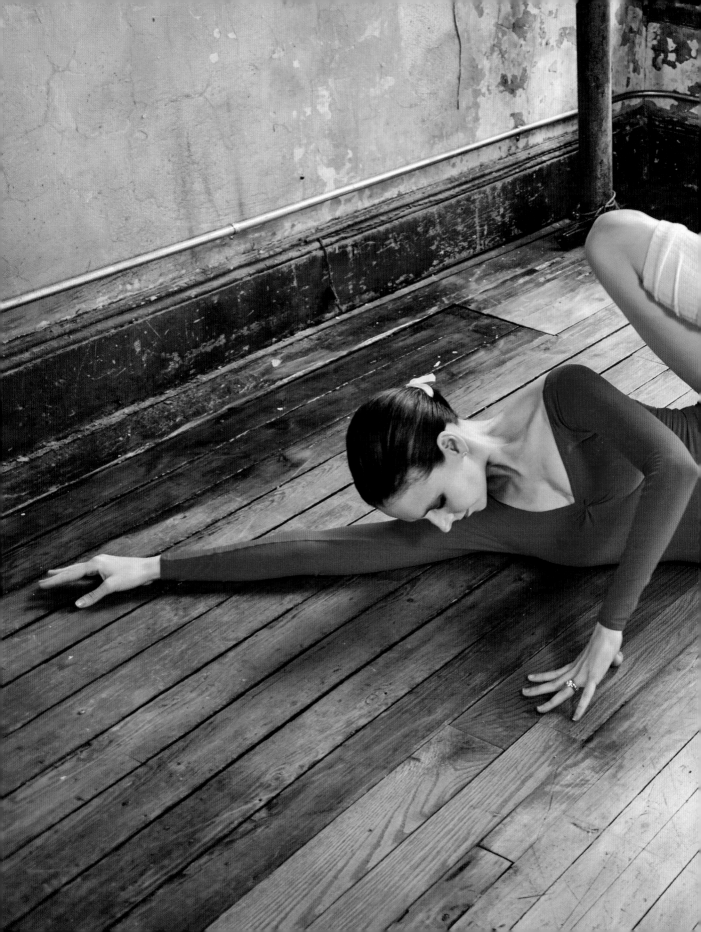

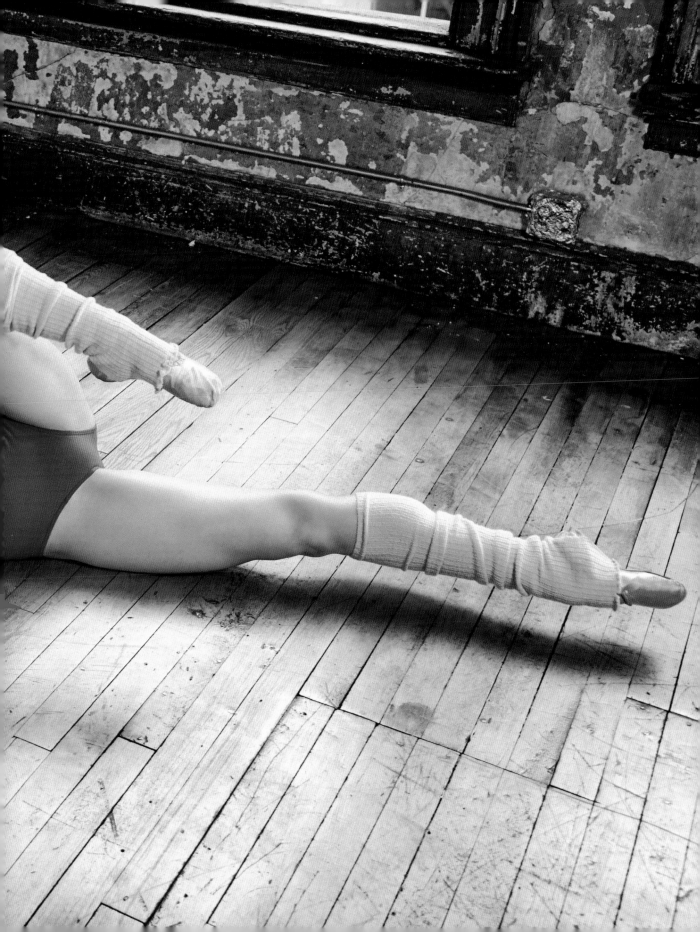

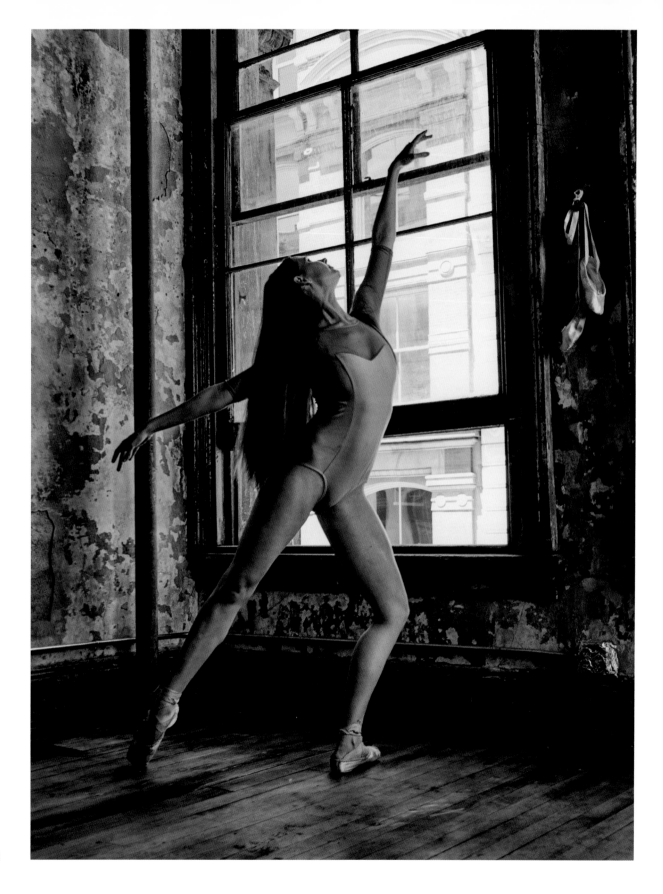

[OPPOSITE] *Plié tendu arabesque.*
[THIS PAGE] Deep front bend.

Dance Principle

A *tendu arabesque* into a front bend both lengthens and strengthens the body. Extend the line in *arabesque* by stretching the limbs long, from the front fingertips to the back toes.

Pro Tip

Imagine a string extending from the fingertips of the hand on the side of the standing leg all the way to the the working toe in *arabesque*. Pull in tight through the abs and core to prevent any arch in the back in *arabesque* and use the stomach muscles to hold and support the body as you move from a front bend back into a *tendu arabesque*.

Fitness Tip

Deep bends to the front work wonders for toning the upper thighs and butt. Combine with a *tendu arabesque* for a deeper burn! Begin with the toes, heels, and knees together in sixth position. Take a deep bend of the knees, lifting the heel of one foot off the ground into a pointed position, reaching low to the ground with the upper body and hands. Hold for eight counts before slowly lifting the upper body up and stretching the lifted foot back long into a *tendu arabesque*. Keep the working knee bent and hold this position for another eight counts, stretch, and change sides.

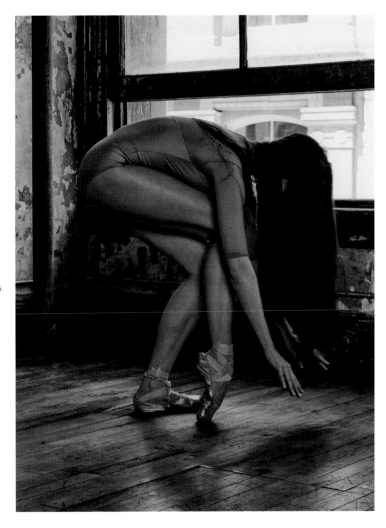

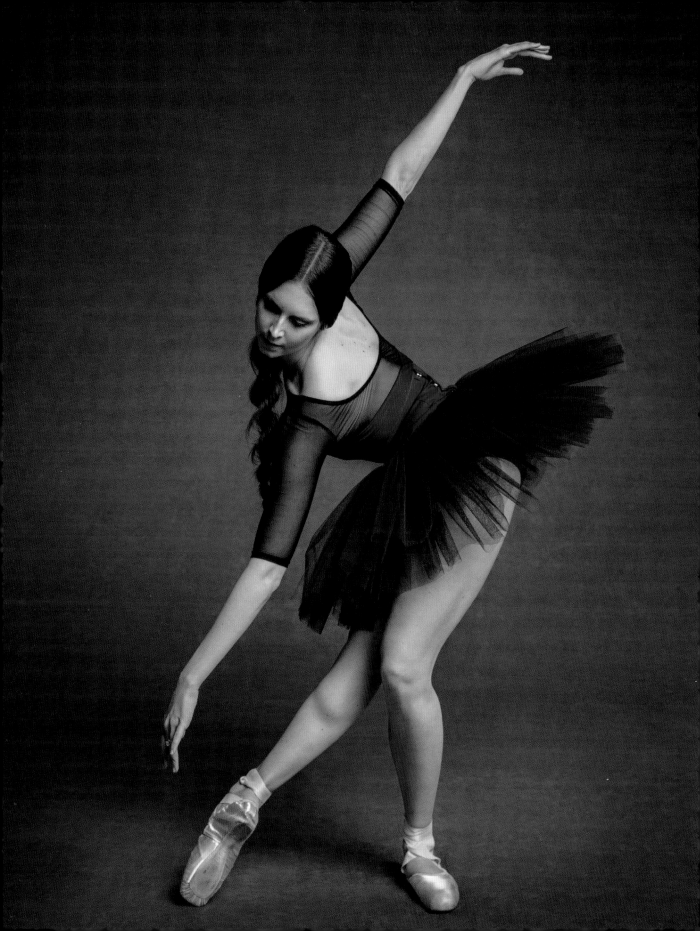

Feet

*T*he feet of a dancer are central to every movement, exhibiting incredible artistry and control. Whether rolling between steps or pushing off and landing from a jump, a dancer's feet both begin and finish almost every step. In ballet, the feet are used both to present the legs to the audience and connect each movement to the ground. Strong feet give a dancer a broader, more powerful dance vocabulary and allow for more precision and better expression. Even a simple walk or run is a dance step onstage—and translating these everyday movements into ballet is some of the most challenging work in dance! A perfectly pointed toe lengthens and extends the legs, providing a culmination to a dancer's line.

For female ballet dancers, pointe shoes lift the foot from a *demi-pointe* (*demi* meaning "half"), with the toes bending and the weight bearing down onto the ball of the foot, to a full *pointe*. The box of a pointe shoe, or toe shoe, supports a dancer's weight *en pointe*, allowing a ballerina to dance, quite literally, on her toes. The result gives lift and length to the line, but not without a cost. Dancing *en pointe* can be excruciatingly painful, depending on the shoes, the dancer's feet, and sometimes just the day. A brand-new pair of pointe shoes is incredibly inflexible and stiff, feeling more like a hard block or brick than a supple slipper. Each new pair of pointe shoes must be specially prepared for performance. Ribbons and elastics are sewn on to secure the shoe on a dancer's foot. Many dancers use elastics around the ankles to hold the arches closer to the sole of the shoe in an effort to maximize a dancer's point. Pointe shoes must also be "broken in" and softened to be made wearable and ready to dance in. Breaking in shoes is a delicate balance. It is important to prepare the shoes for dancing and allow the hard inner shank to bend with the pointing of the toes without making them too soft to dance on.

The process of "breaking in" a new pair of shoes and even wrapping and protecting the feet against blisters is incredibly personal to each dancer. I like to feel the floor, to a certain extent, when dancing *en pointe*. I remove a few nails from the shank of my pointe shoes, step on the box to soften the *demi-pointe*, and bend the upper half of the shank, sometimes even cutting the top quarter or third of the shank off the shoe to make the arch more pliable. Before I slip my pointe shoes on, I stop to prepare my feet to dance *en pointe*. I wrap strips of paper towels around my individual toes and the balls of my feet to prevent blisters and friction. This provides a lightweight barrier between my feet and my shoes that absorbs sweat as my feet warm up and the shoes begin to soften and break in.

While Ballet Beautiful workouts do not require *pointe* work, strong feet can help all of us prevent injury and better strengthen our legs, body, and core. Whether dancing on or off pointe, simple conditioning exercises like pointing and flexing the toes and feet builds strength to add support for better expression of the legs and control. Basic foot work rolling through the toes and feet from a full point to a flat foot is a terrific preparation for jumping along with more advanced standing exercises and center work in a ballet class or onstage. *Relevés* on *demi-* or full *pointe* practiced at the barre or even against a wall (or piano!) can then be repeated in the center to build additional strength and stability through the arches.

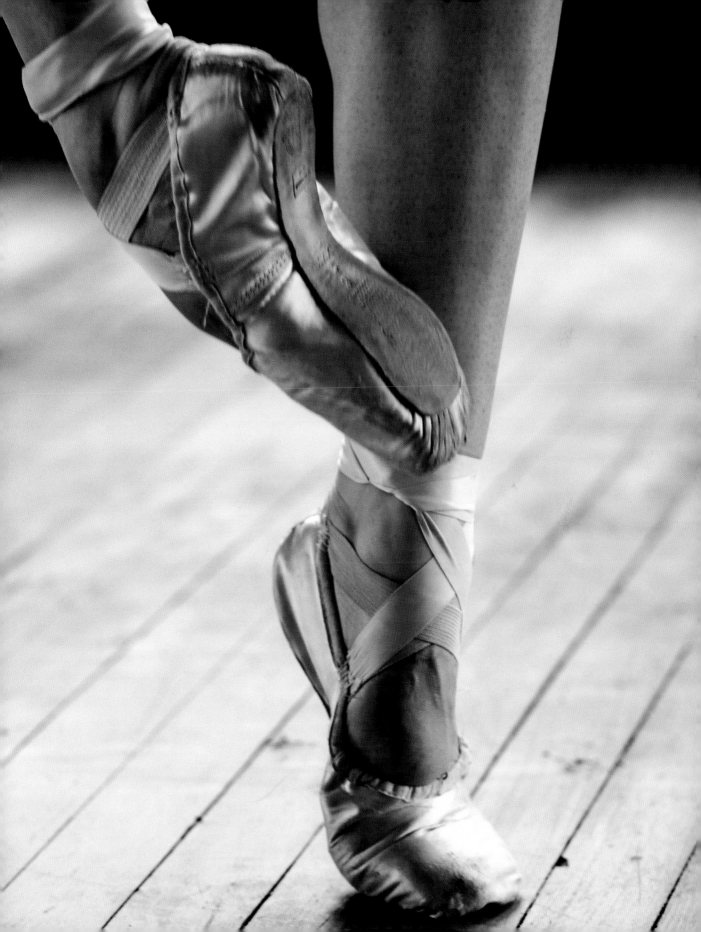

[PREVIOUS PAGES] *Relevé sur le cou-de-pied.*

A *relevé* is a lift onto a *demi-* or full *pointe*. Sur le *cou-de-pied* means "on the neck of the foot," describing the position of the foot rather than an actual movement, with the working toe beside the ankle and the heel at the base of the calf. The toe can be placed in front of the leg at the front of the ankle (pictured), at the back, or in a wrapped position with the heel in the front of the ankle and the toe wrapping around the "neck" of the foot.

Dance Principle
*Relevé*s on *demi-pointe* warm up the feet, preparing the body for a wide range of motion.

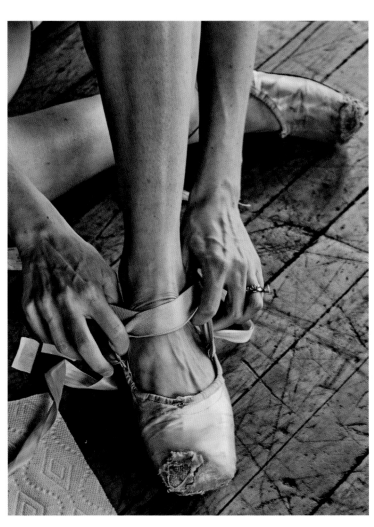

[THIS PAGE + OPPOSITE] Every dancer has a different approach to preparing both their feet and shoes to dance *en pointe.*

[OPPOSITE]
Dance Principle
Ribbons and elastics are sewn onto pointe shoes to hold the shoes to a dancer's feet through a whirlwind of movement. Crossing elastic bands across the arch brings the arch closer to the shank, or inner sole, of the shoe, improving a dancer's pointe and making the shoes feel tighter and more secure.

[THIS PAGE]
Pro Tip
Wrapping paper towels around the toes and balls of the feet creates a lightweight, protective layer for the feet inside a pair of pointe shoes, preventing friction and blisters when dancing *en pointe.* Paper towels break down and absorb sweat as the feet warm up and the shoes begin to soften.

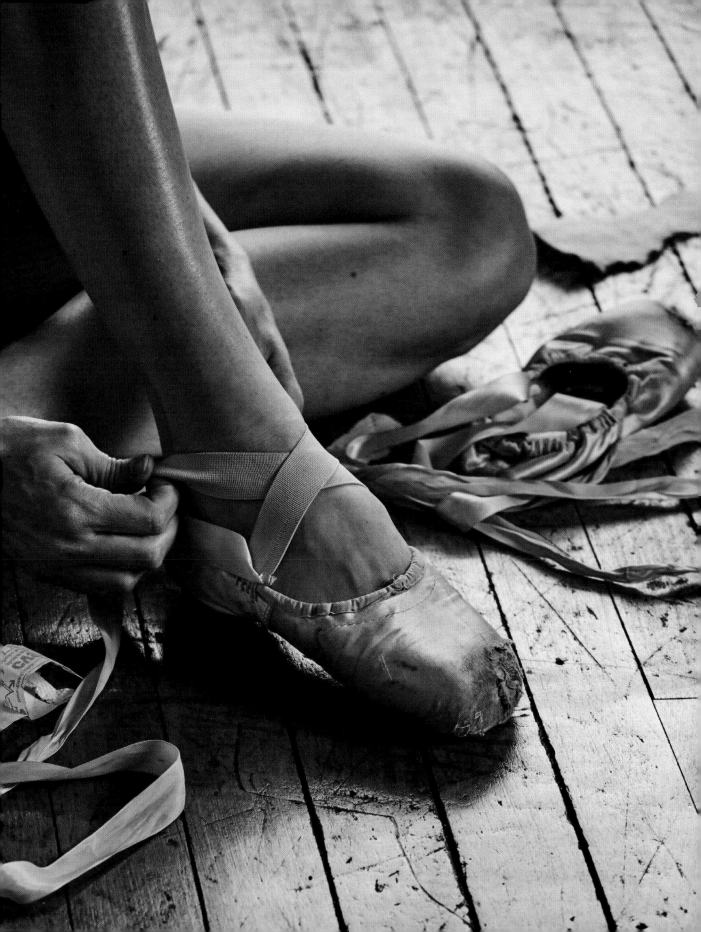

Pushing the arches over *en pointe* helps to prepare both the shoes and feet to point at their fullest.

Fitness Tip
A lift on *demi-pointe* warms up the feet. From a seated position, bend both knees and lift the feet up onto *demi-pointe*, pushing the arches forward. Hold this position for eight counts. For a more challenging stretch, repeat this stretch while lifting the hips. Hold eight counts.

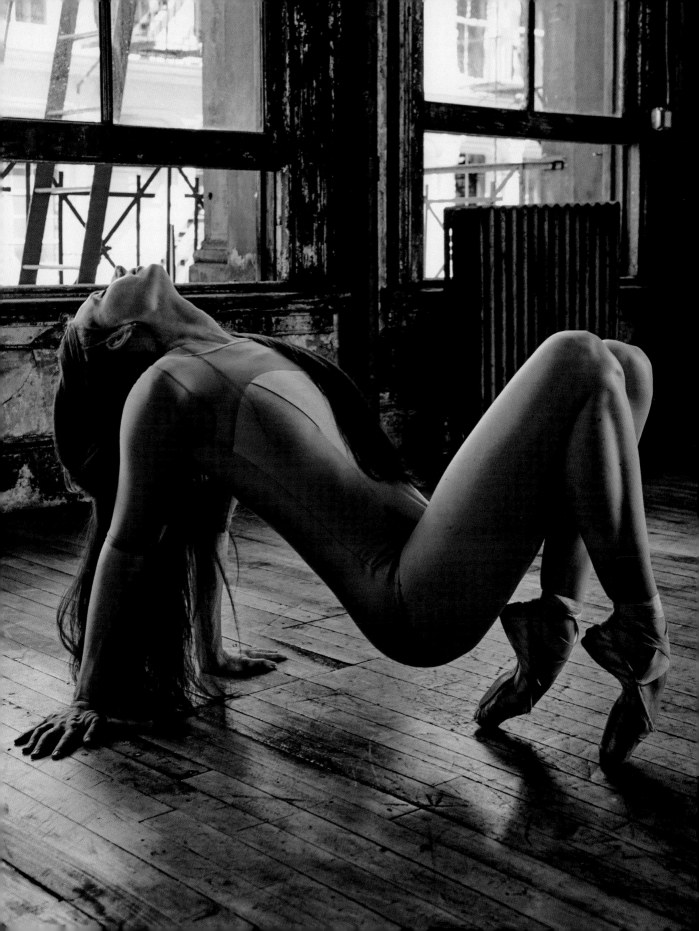

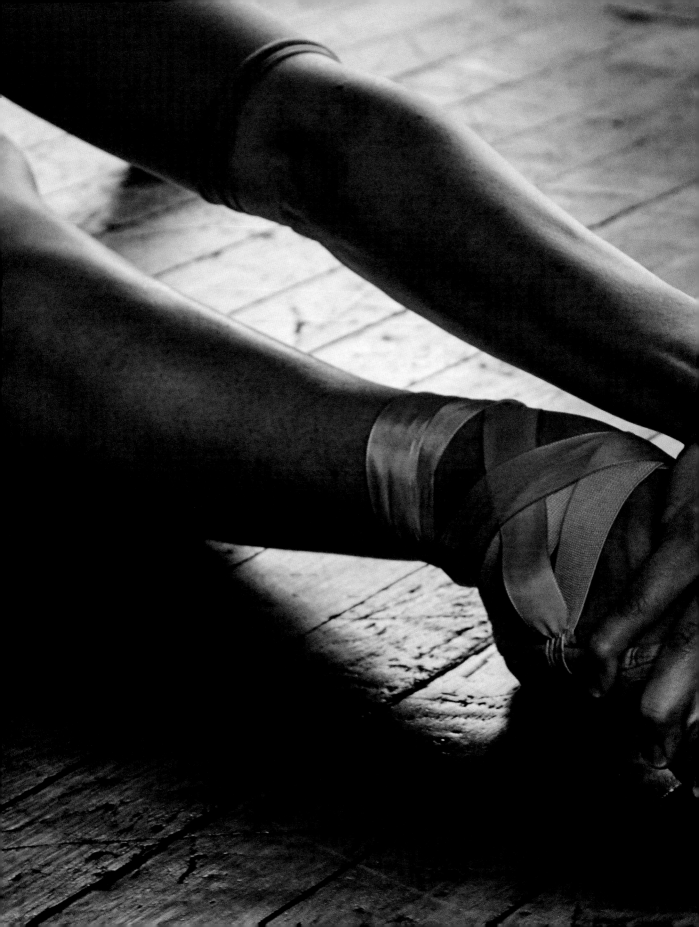

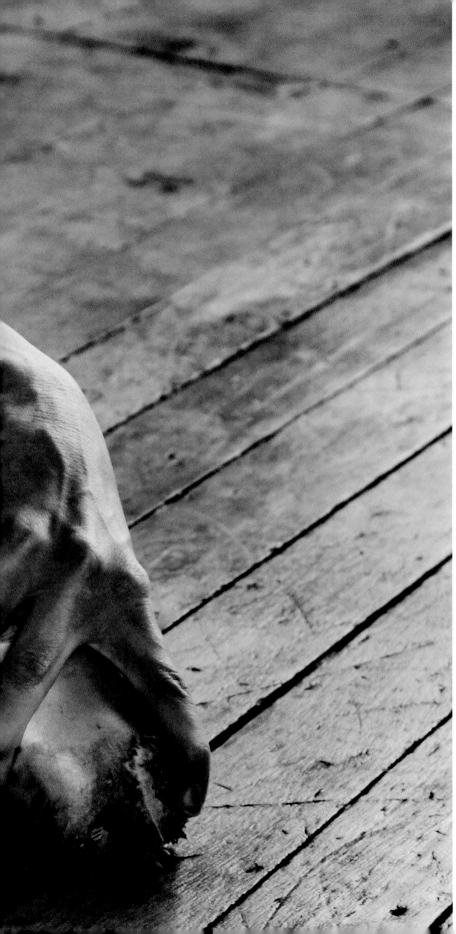

Finding the perfect pointe.

Dance Principle
Warming up the feet is an essential part of preparing the body to dance. Once the shoes are on the feet, the ribbons are tied along the inside of the ankle and tucked into place. A few stitches at the ankle where the ribbons are tucked in hold any loose pieces in place when a dancer is on stage.

Pro Tip
Bending the shoe to the arch while pointing the foot helps mold pointe shoes to a dancer's foot and maximize the pointe.

Fitness Tip
Prevent cramping in the arches and feet with a ballet warm-up. In a seated position, place one hand along the top and one along the inside of the top of the arch in the center of the foot. Massage the arches gently with both hands while moving the feet from a flexed to a pointed position, moving the hands slowly toward the toes.

55

The warm-up. "Rolling through" the balls of the feet warms and prepares the feet and shoes to dance *en pointe*.

Dance Principle
Pushing both arches over onto pointe helps to break in a pair of pointe shoes.

Pro Tip
Use a wall or barre to balance when warming up the feet and breaking in new shoes.

Fitness Tip
This dance-based warm up for the feet is the perfect pre-cardio prep. Move one foot at a time from flat, to demi, to a full pointe with a light pumping motion, alternating feet each time. Repeat for two sets of eight with a fluid movement.

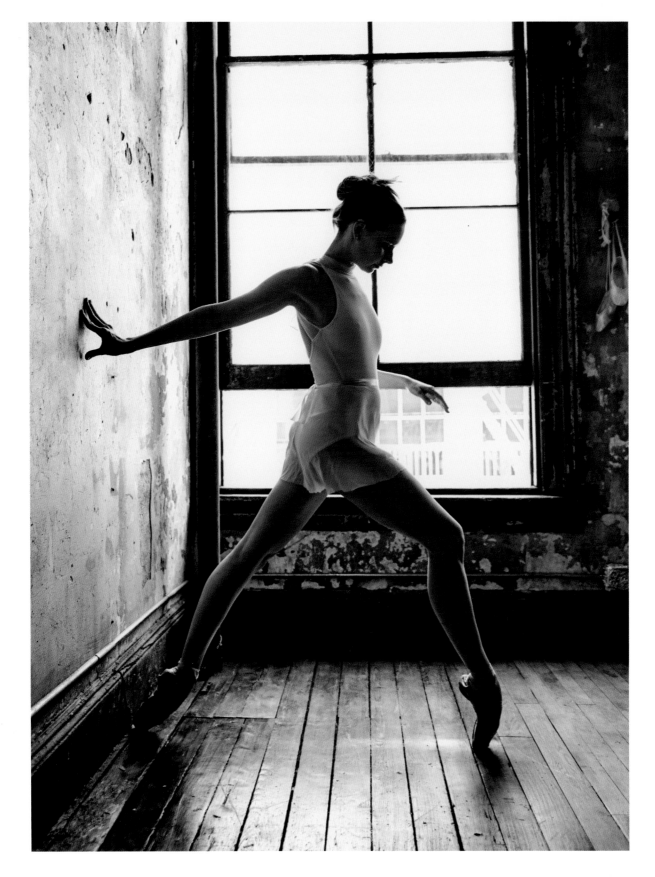

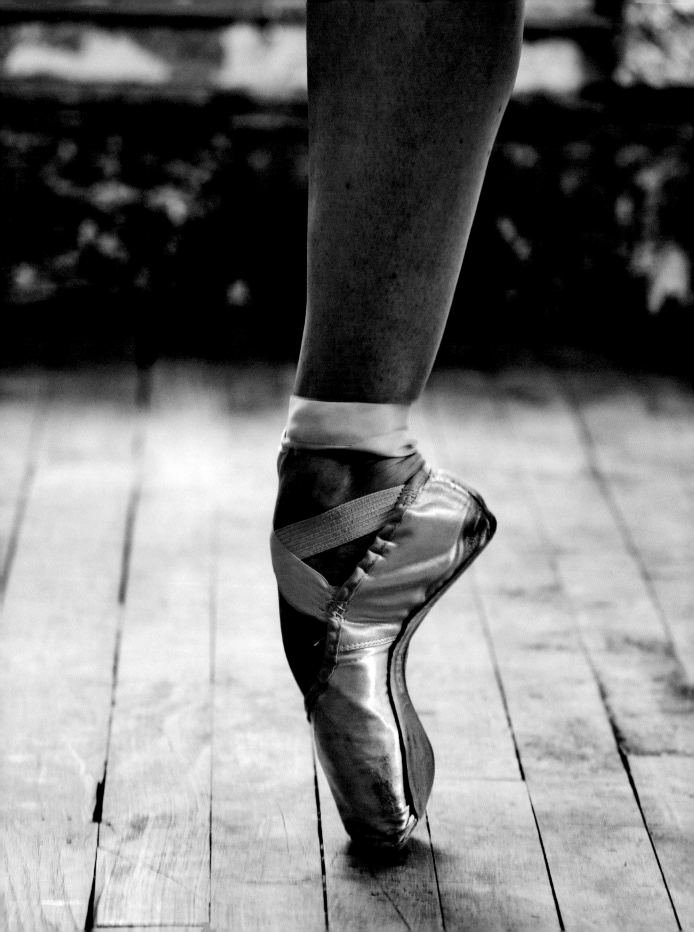

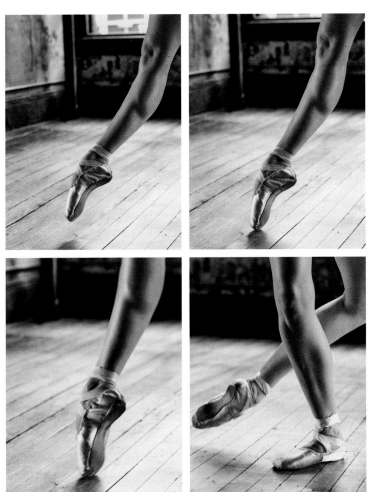

[THIS PAGE + OPPOSITE] A fully pointed foot extends and completes the lines of the legs.

Fitness Tip

Add a pointed toe to your next workout to strengthen and condition the tops of the feet, arches, and calves. Bring the heels together and open the toes in a relaxed first position. Point the foot and lift the leg into the air to forty-five degrees. Hold for two sets of eight. Lower the foot and repeat on the other side.

[FOLLOWING PAGES] *Relevé sur le cou-de-pied* ("on the 'neck' of the foot").

Pro Tip

Lift high through the arches, taking care not to roll or pronate the feet to build strength and stability through the feet and ankles.

Fitness Tip

Relevés on one foot strengthen and tone muscles in both the feet and calves. Lift one foot off the floor with a pointed toe, turning out from the hip. Place the toe at either the front of the ankle or in a wrapped position (pictured) around the ankle of the standing leg. Using a barre, chair, or wall for balance, slowly lift the standing leg onto *demi-pointe*. Lower the foot to flat and repeat, two sets of eight, then change sides.

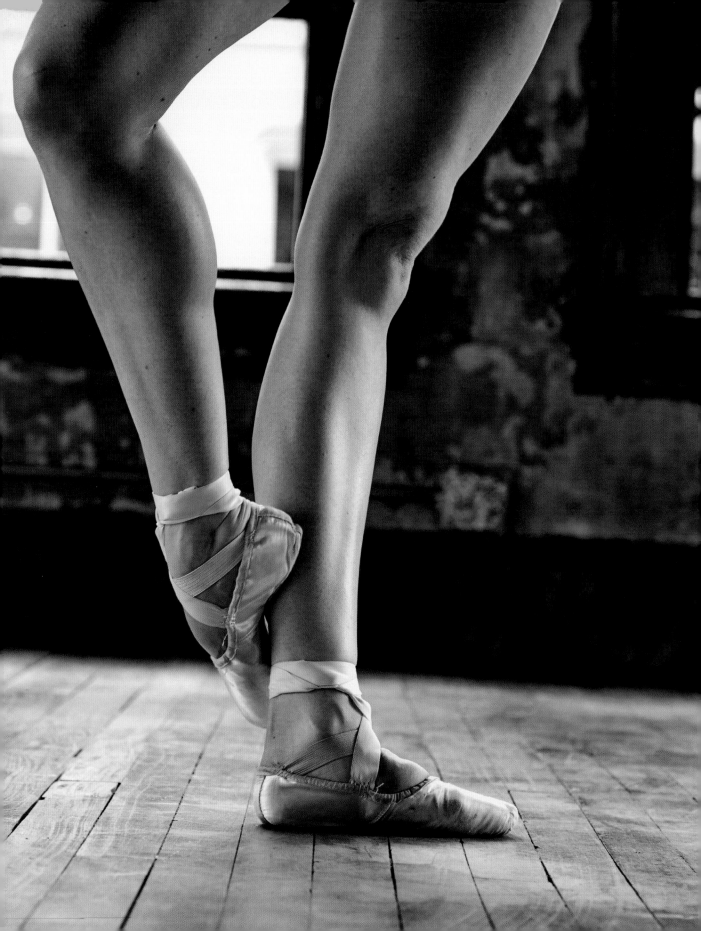

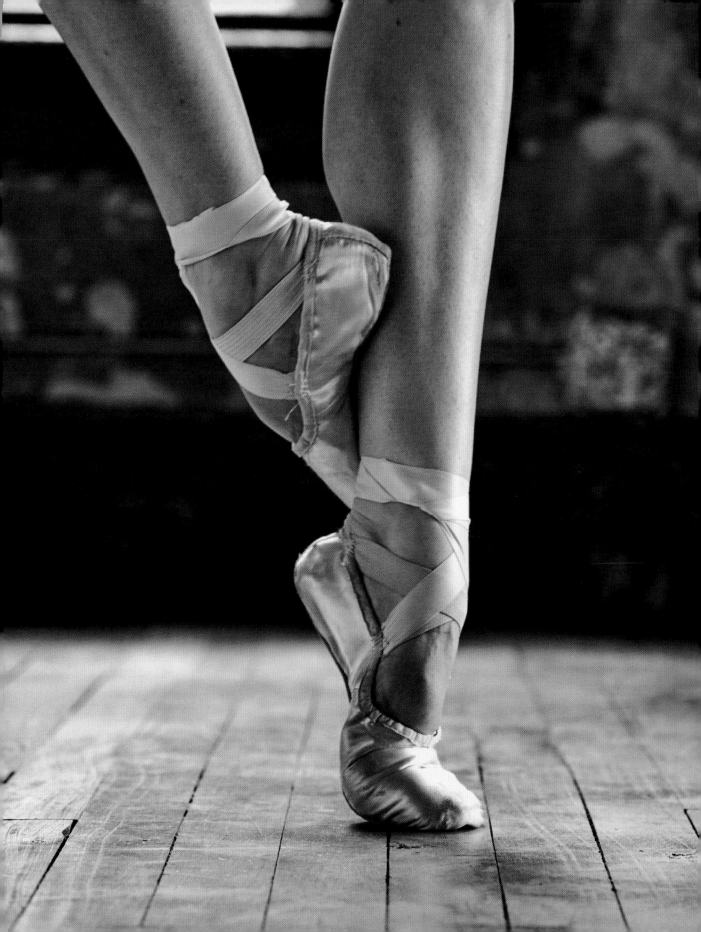

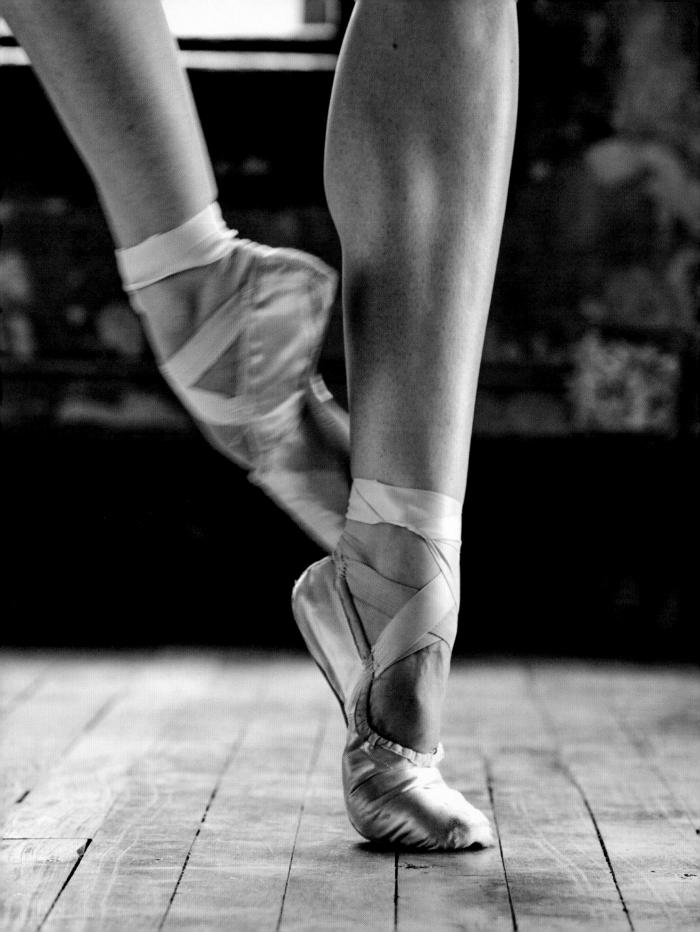

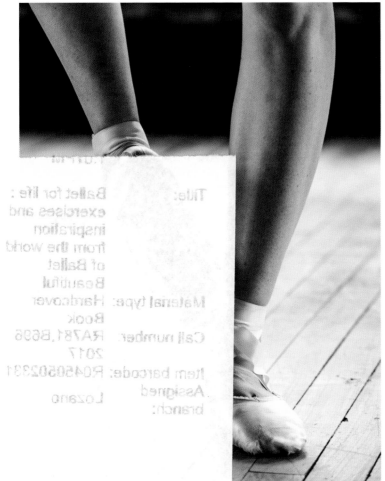

[THIS PAGE + OPPOSITE] *Petit battement à terre* and *sur la demi-pointe.*

Dance Principle

Petits battements, meaning "small beats," engage inner thighs and develop control through the feet and lower legs.

Pro Tip

A slight "wing" of the foot, a position where the toes bend slightly back with the heel to the front, allows for better speed and form in a series of *petits battements*.

[FOLLOWING PAGES, FROM LEFT] Fifth position with the feet flat, and on *demi-pointe.*

Dance Principle

Fifth position is the most advanced of the five positions of the feet. When working in fifth, line up the feet, toe to heel and heel to toe, turning the legs out from the hips and lifting through the arches of the feet. On *relevé,* the same basic position is repeated with the feet lifted onto a half or full pointe.

Fitness Tip

A simple *plié relevé* in fifth position tones the calves, inner thighs, and butt while strengthening the arches and feet. Hold on to a barre or wall for extra support. Cross the feet toe to heel. Bend both knees into a *demi plié,* leaving the heels on the floor. Pull in with the abs and spring up onto *demi-pointe* on both feet, crossing the ankles as the legs and feet move to fifth position *en demi-pointe.* Repeat for one to two sets of eight, and then stretch and change sides.

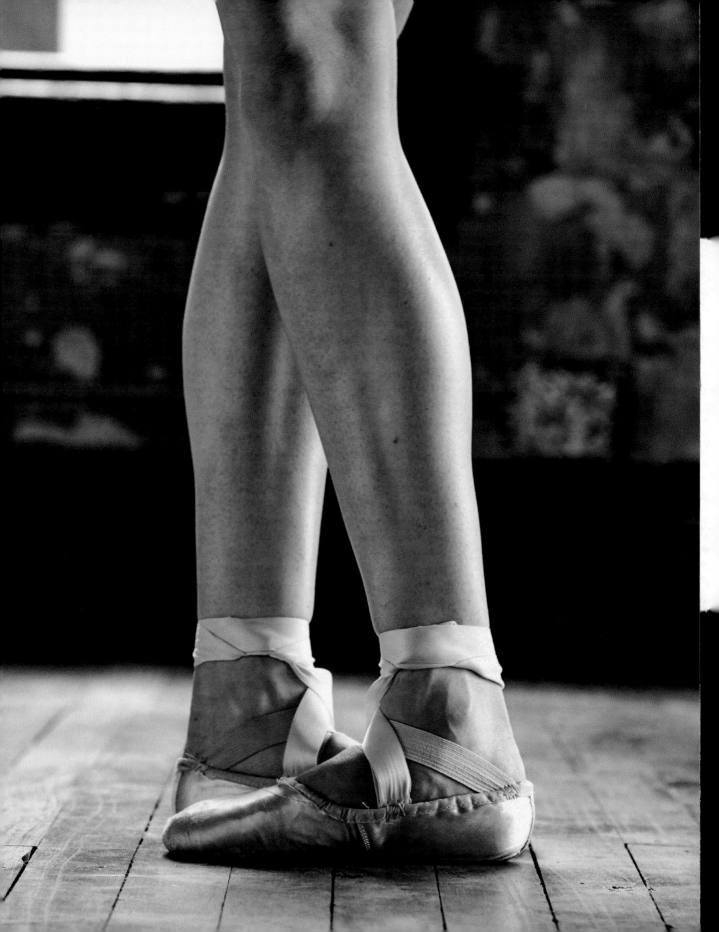

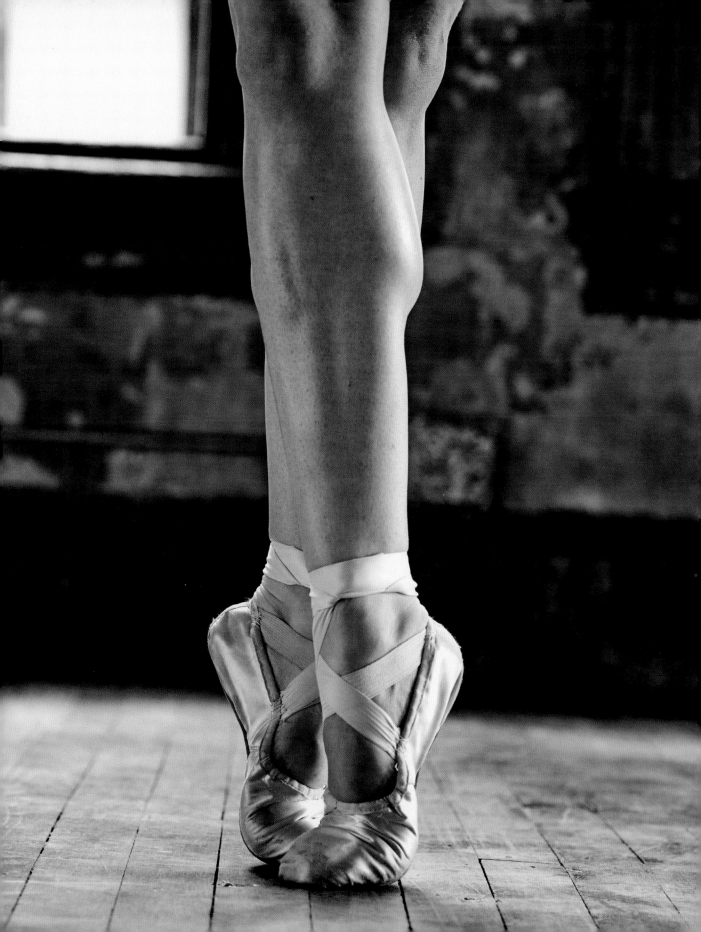

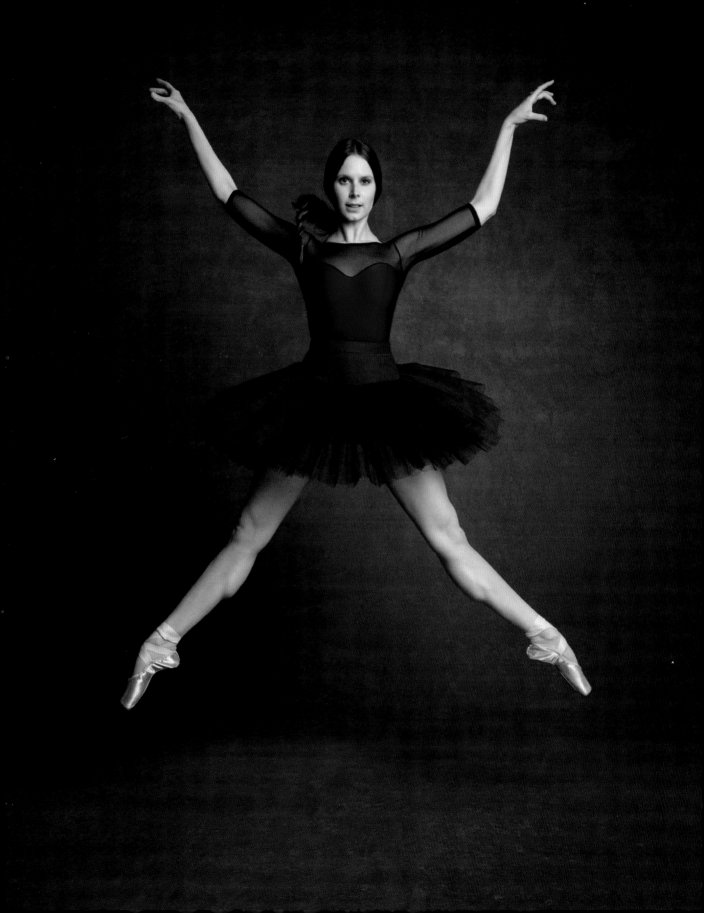

I . 3

Center

*D*ancers engage their abdominals in almost every movement they perform, making even the simplest ballet step an abdominal workout, too. All a dancer's movement originates from her center. This constant pulling in and engagement of the abs, whether performing a simple port de bras, plié, *or a more complicated* grand battement *strengthens the core while whittling the waist, building a center that is strong and lean. In dance the core is the center of balance. It is the key to turning, jumping, and, above all, to control.*

As a young dancer, I was extremely flexible but my body was relatively weak. Focusing on strengthening my center helped me develop the muscles needed to hold my extensions, complete my turns, and power through jumps. Having a strong center helps with balance, too. If you are struggling with balance, pulling in the stomach engages the abs and helps to immediately stabilize. This trick is helpful for choreography and center work and is particularly useful when it comes to turns. Never was this more apparent to me than when dancing on raked, or inclined, stages overseas on tour with New York City Ballet. In the United States we are used to dancing on a flat stage with the audience tiered in stadium-style seating. Many an older theater overseas, however, has a raked or angled stage while the seating for the audience is on a flat floor. For a dancer, the difference is dramatic. Imagine dancing and performing *en pointe* on a hill! Adjusting can be nerve-wracking as the center of balance is completely different for each individual dancer and stage. Some of my most powerful and memorable performances with New York City Ballet occurred overseas—and having to adapt my performance to a rake in a theater like the Mariinsky in Saint Petersburg added anxiety, intensifying the experience. I vividly remember the elation I felt on smoothly completing the dizzying *piqué* turn passage in Balanchine's Serenade onstage in Russia. Thank goodness for that ballet core!

Because the abdominal muscles are so central to every movement, they are the perfect place to begin each workout. Once the abdominal muscles are warm and working, pulling the stomach in tight and thinking of closing the top of the ribs together to prevent any arch in the back helps to keep the abs engaged through every exercise. One of my favorite visuals is imagining "pulling" the belly button to the spine. This not only keeps the abdominal muscles as a whole engaged and working deep within the core, but also especially engages the lower abs, which are notoriously difficult to target. Imagine someone taking a photo of you in a bathing suit just as you lift and twist the abs during mat work. This visual cues us to pull the stomach in tight, thereby engaging the abdominals from the lowest to the highest point in the core. Simple twisting movements through the sides also work the oblique muscles in the abdominal wall, strengthening the core and toning the stomach and waist.

Battement à la seconde.

Dance Principle
Grands (large) *battements* require power and control. In a *battement*, the kick both targets and originates from the core.

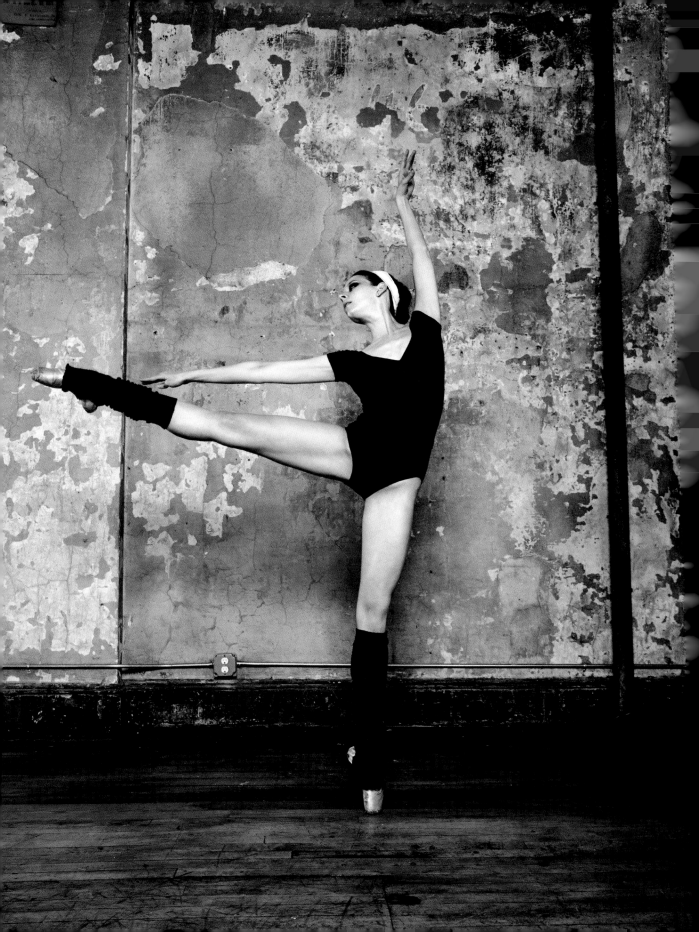

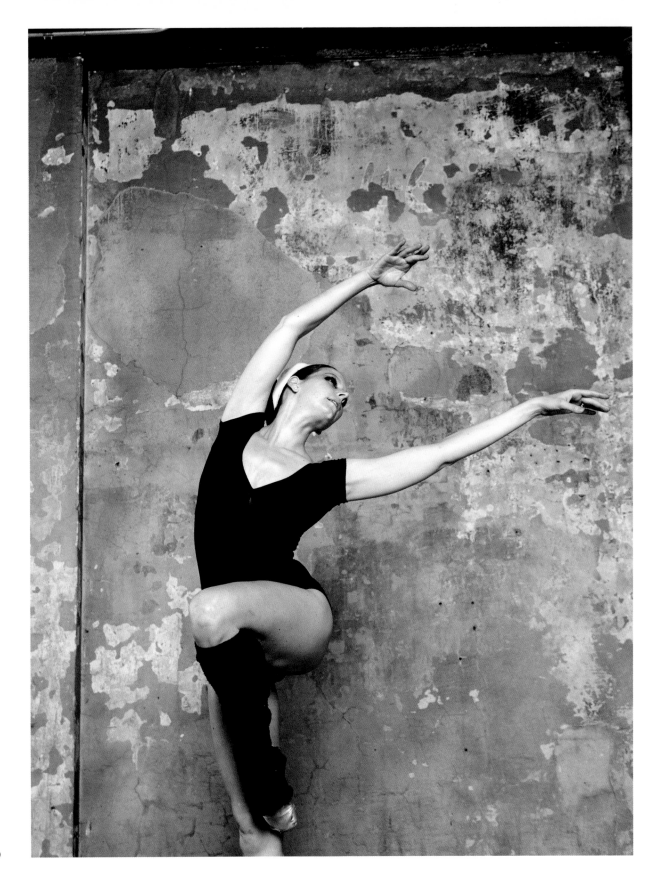

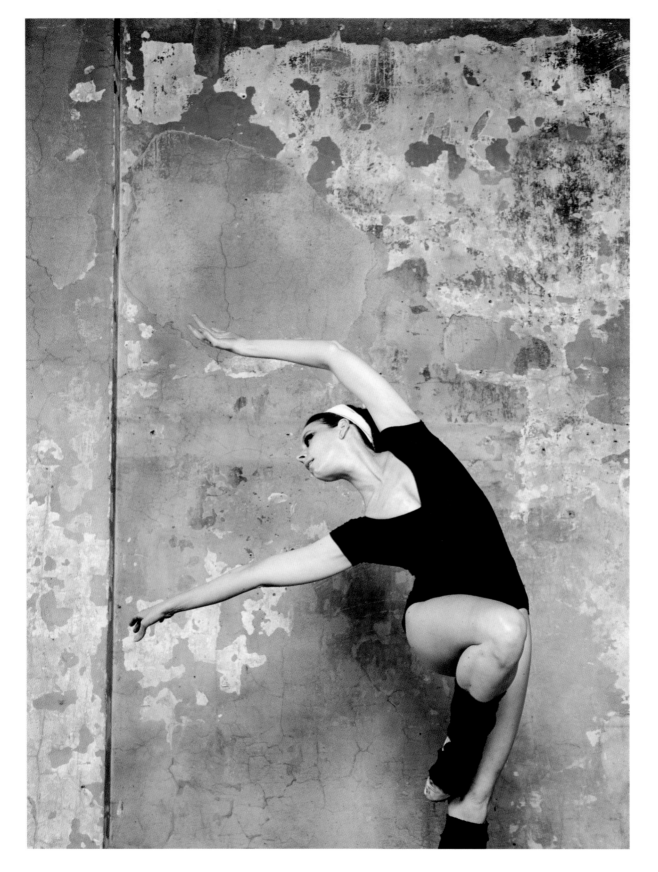

[PREVIOUS PAGES] *Passé* in parallel with a lyrical bend through the waist.

Dance Principle

The opposition between the lifted knee and upper body in this position strengthens and challenges the abs.

Fitness Tip

A *cambré* (meaning "arch") to the side targets the abs while sculpting the waist. Beginning in sixth position (toes together, heels together), lift one foot up into a *passé* parallel, bringing the working toe to standing knee. Lift up and over with the upper body, pulling in tight through the abs in the same direction as the lifted knee. Hold for two to four counts, lower and change sides.

[OPPOSITE] *Plié tendu en avant*: the standing knee is bent with the working leg stretched long to the front. A slight bend through the waist engages and tones the core.

Dance Principle

The abdominals connect the movement, from the fingertips to the toes. Pull up and in with the stomach as you twist through the waist, extending the front toe long.

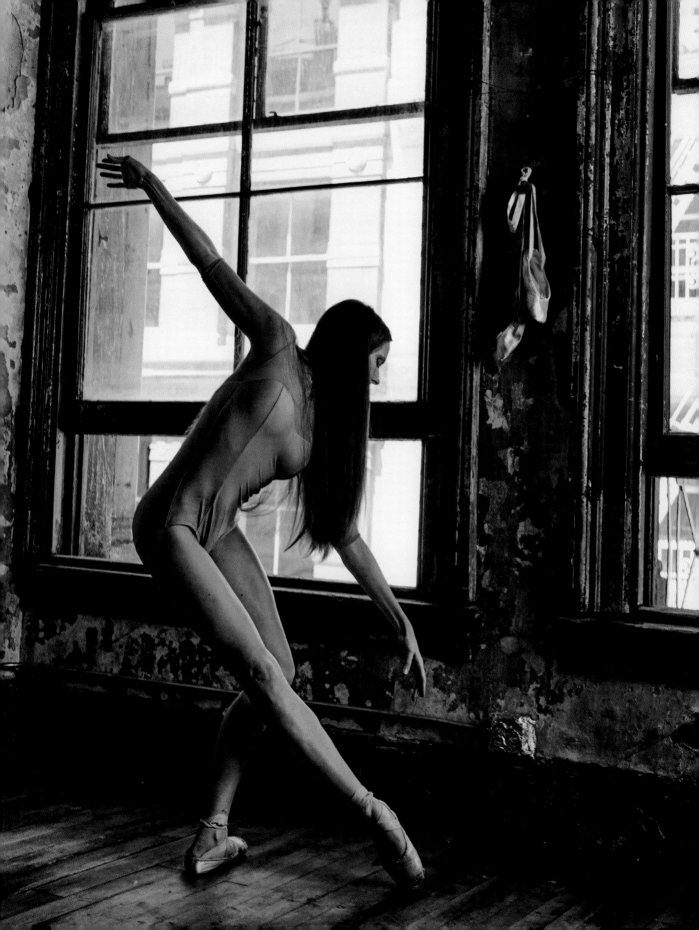

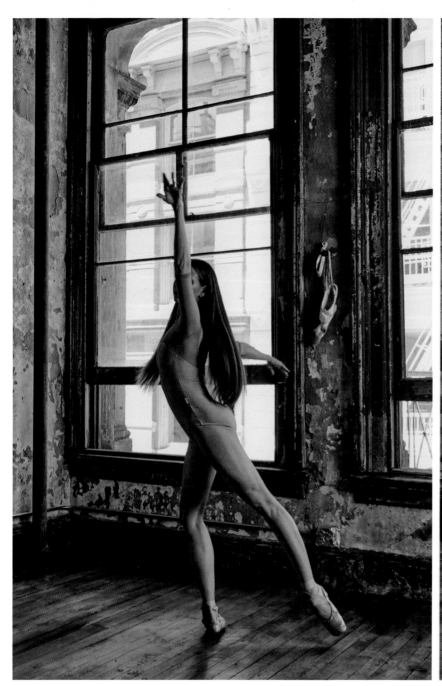

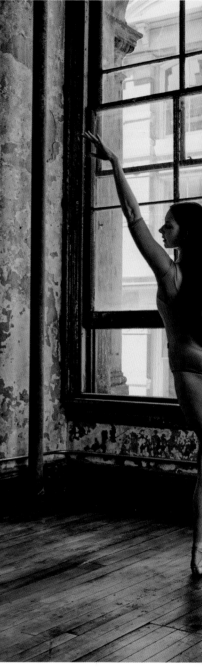

Pivot turns in *arabesque* require control in the legs, feet, and core.

Dance Principle
Lift the heel slightly off the floor to pivot (turn) on the ball of the foot, keeping the ribcage closed and the abs pulled in tight.

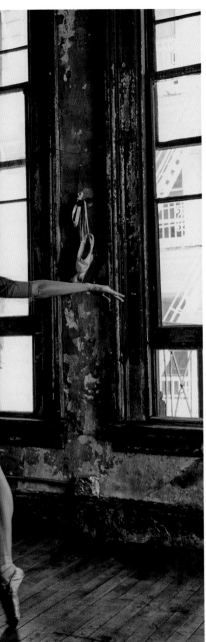

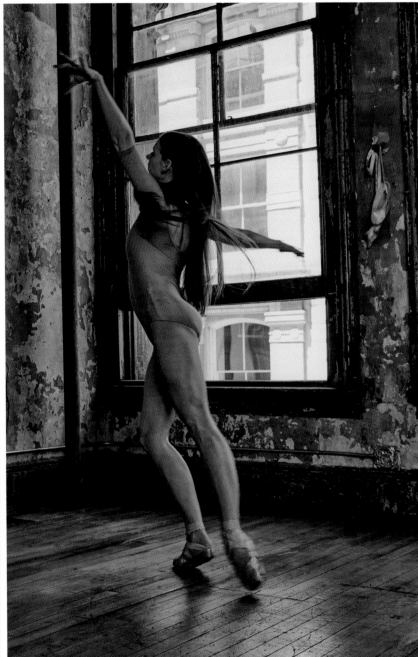

Fitness Tip

Start small, focusing on standing abdominal work for the upper body before adding in a turn with the legs. Begin by keeping the feet still in a *tendu arabesque* and turning the upper body twenty degrees, toward the standing leg, pulling in tight with the abs. As your body begins to feel more at ease with the movement, pick up the heel slightly and turn ten to twenty degrees to start, working your way up to 180 degrees and then a full 360-degree turn over time. Repeat on the other side.

75

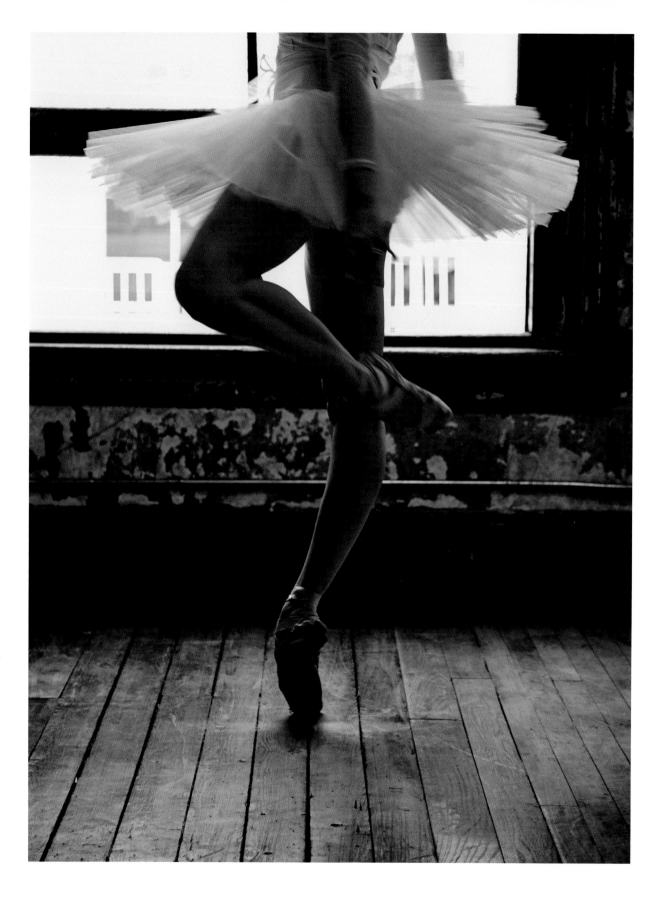

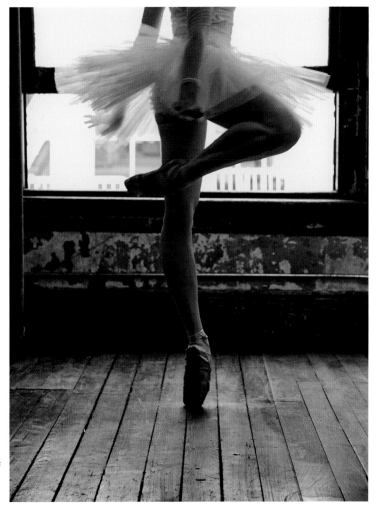

[THIS PAGE + OPPOSITE] *Piqué* turns *en pointe*.

Dance Principle
When turning *en pointe*, abdominal strength and control is key.

Pro Tip
Pull in tight through the ribs and waist and lift through the hips for extra control.

Fitness Tip
*Piqué passé*s at the barre or using a wall or chair are a great introductory step for more advanced dance steps like *piqué* turns. Step up onto a straight working leg with the back leg bent into a *passé*, working toe to the back of the knee. Lift to *demi-pointe* to challenge the abs and engage the lower calves or keep the foot flat to maintain the focus on the working leg and butt. Repeat for two sets of eight, and then change sides.

[FOLLOWING PAGES] Almost every movement in ballet originates from a dancer's center and core. Abdominal exercises on the mat or floor warm up and strengthen the core.

Fitness Tip
Improve your center of balance and strength with ballet-inspired abdominal work. Pull the stomach in tight, belly button to spine, to target and engage the lower abs. Lift the upper body off the floor, bending one knee in toward the chest while extending the other leg straight to the front, keeping the leg and foot off the floor. Hold for eight counts and then change sides. Repeat the complete movement four to six times.

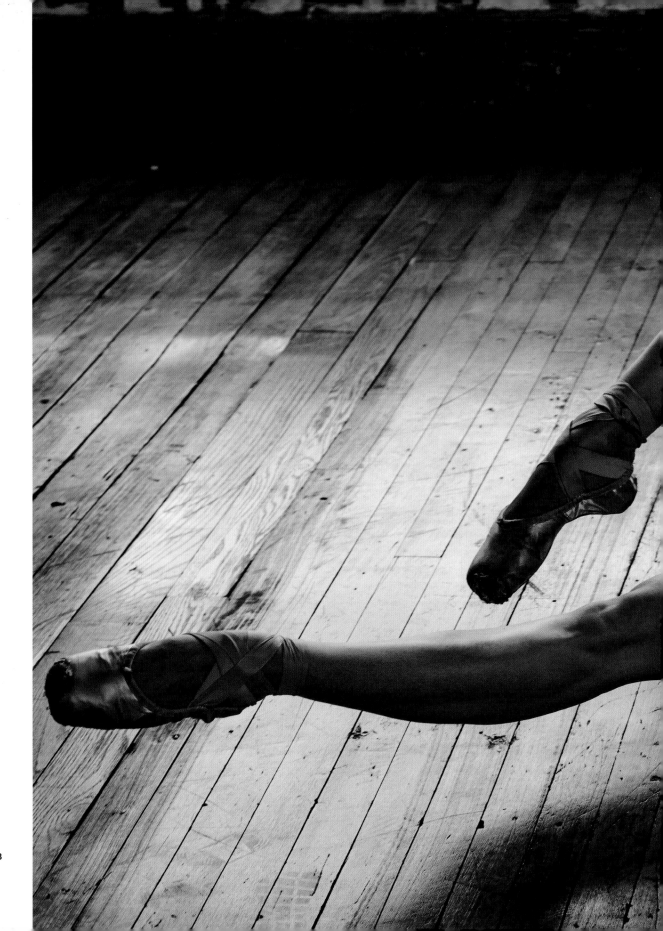

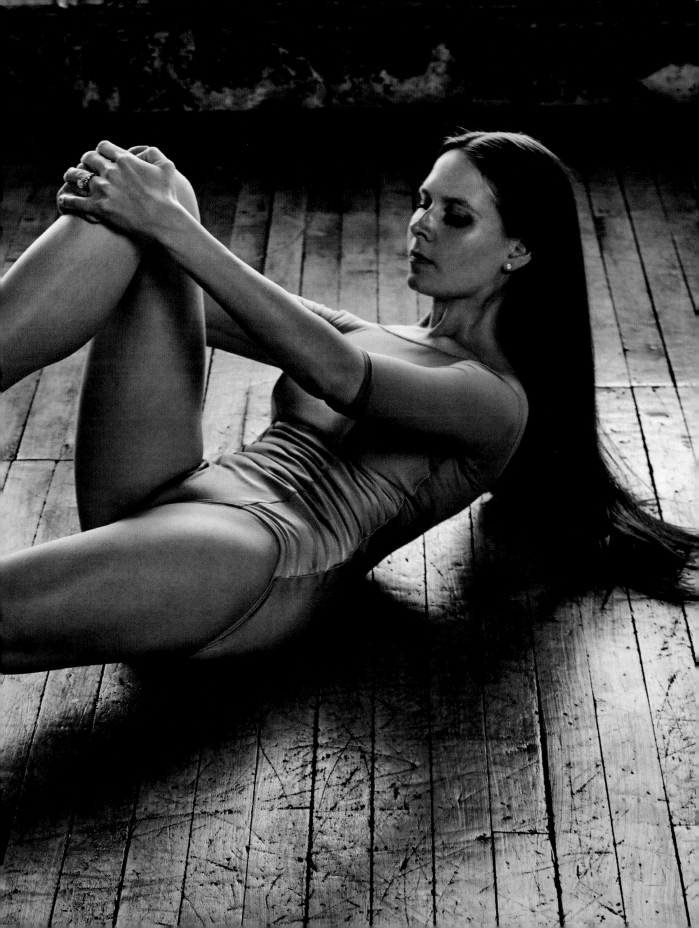

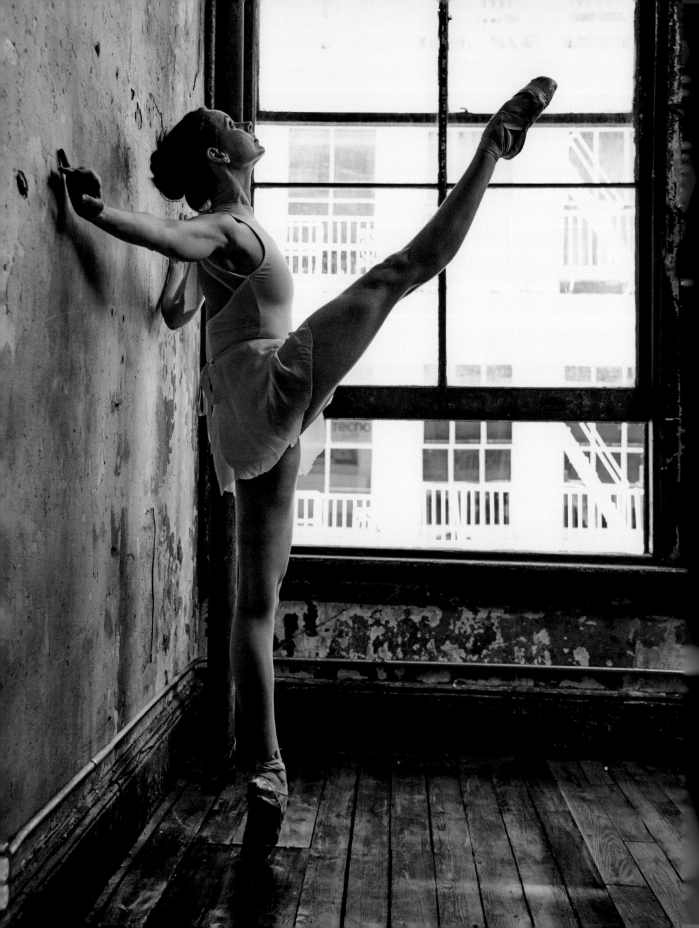

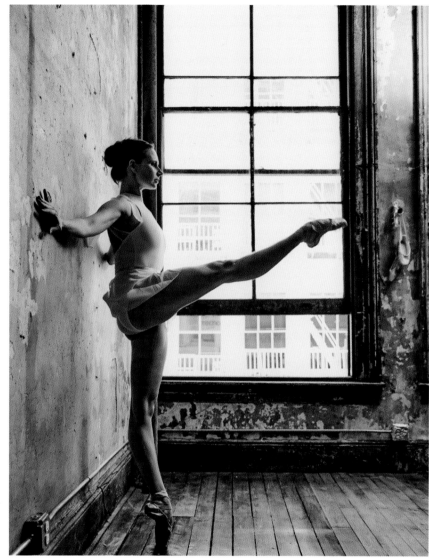

Développé devant en pointe. Développé means "to develop," and a *développé* is an adagio movement, or slow movement, that requires terrific strength and control. The working leg moves from *cou-de-pied* through *retiré passé* and into an *attitude* before stretching long into a *développé* to the front. May be performed to the front (*devant*), to the side (*à la seconde*), or to the back (*derrière*).

Dance Principle
Strong abdominals help to lift and extend the legs, helping a dancer to hold the position.

Fitness Tip
Don't worry about the height of the leg, focus on proper form rather than extension. Begin by practicing a *développé* at forty-five degrees, opening the legs from the hips, and slowly lift the toe and working leg from *cou-de-pied* to *passé* and then stretch the leg to the front. Stretch and change sides.

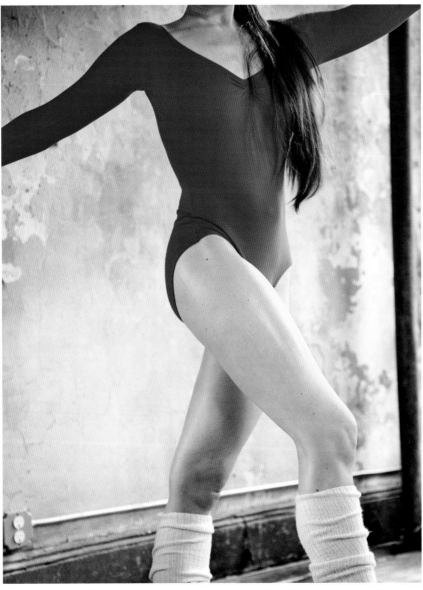

Core twist.

Dance Principle
Opposition between the arms and legs adds challenge and complexity to a basic twisting movement.

Fitness Tip
Begin standing with one knee bent and one straight, twisting the upper body to the side, toward the working knee. Pull the abs in, belly button to spine, as you bend the standing knee, deepening the twist through the upper body. Hold and pulse lightly through the upper body, deepening the twist in the waist for two sets of eight. Stretch and repeat the other side.

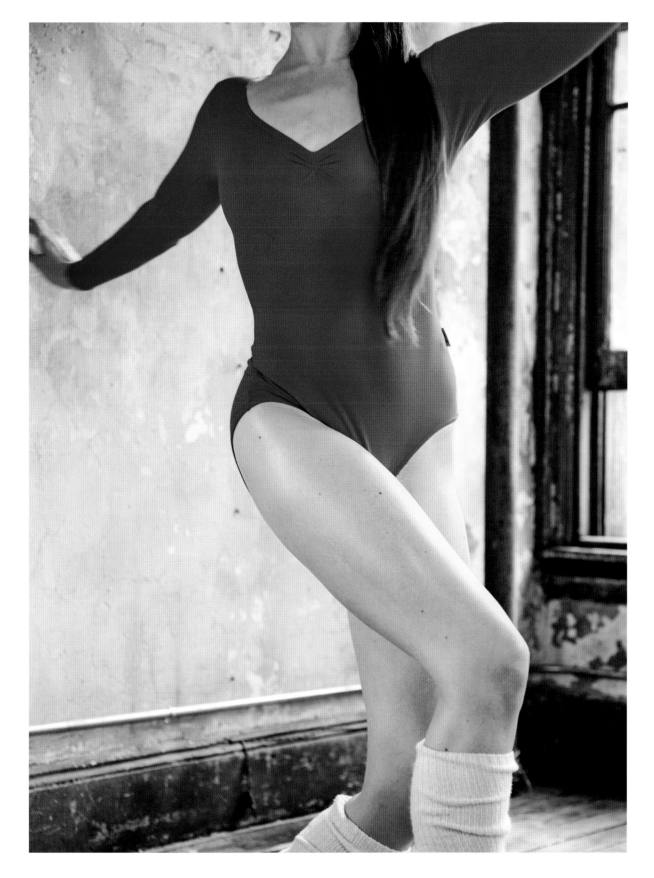

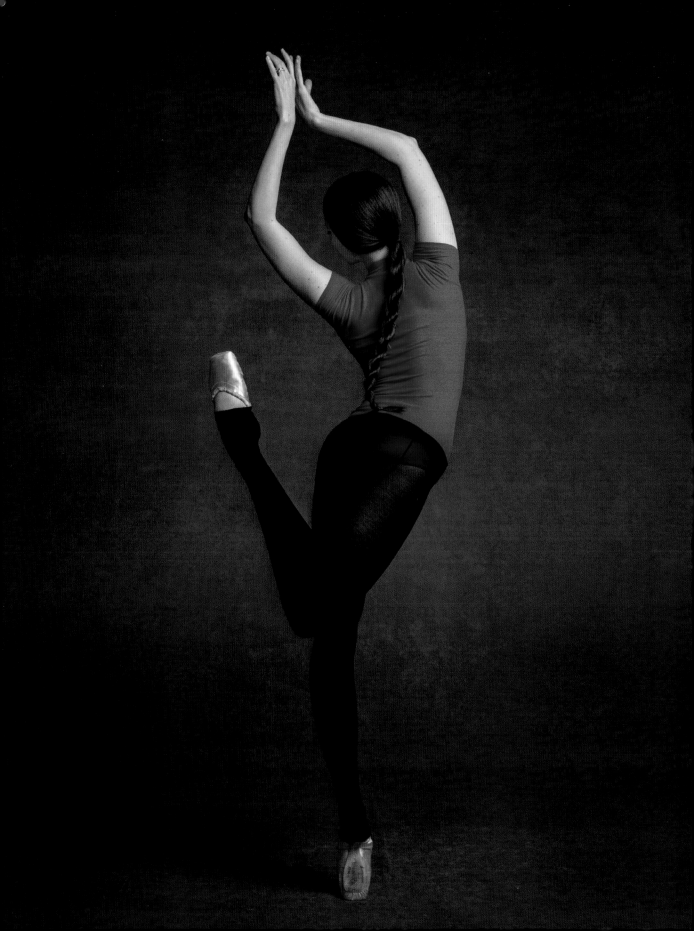

I . 4

Derrière

Much like the abdominal muscles, dancers use their gluteus muscles in almost every movement, beginning at the barre. The base position for most barre and center work is a very active one. The body is lifted, the chest is open, and the legs are stretched and elongated, with abdominal muscles engaged. The hips are straight and the butt is squeezed and lifted.

For non-dancers, this neutral position can feel very "tucked," almost as if the hips are being thrust under and forward. There should not be any bend in the hips or arch in the back, but rather a straight line from the thighs to the waist. This basic position alone is a workout, engaging the glutes, abs, and muscles in the upper body, too. Beginning with this active starting position, a classical ballet class moves through a proper warm-up at the barre starting with *pliés*, *tendus*, and *relevés* followed by more advanced movements like *rond de jambes*, *arabesques*, *fondues*, *attitudes*, *grands battements*, and *adagio* work, all of which engage, lift and tone the derrière as the body warms up. This progression of movements is then repeated in the center of the room as the dancers execute another series of *pliés*, *tendus*, and *adagio* work, this time without any support, along with *pirouettes*, *waltzes*, *petit and grand allegro*, further working the derrière.

When I left New York City Ballet and took a short break from training, I was dismayed to see my butt quickly flatten out without this daily routine. But as soon as I picked up with my workout again and began developing Ballet Beautiful, my derrière perked right up too. Glutes exercises are some of the most popular of the Ballet Beautiful program because they deliver terrific results, lifting and sculpting without bulking.

Ballet Beautiful mimics the natural progression of movement in classical ballet training that engages and targets the glutes. Exercises like our targeted Ballet Lunges, which are inspired by the kneeling passage in the "Waltz" scene in Balanchine's iconic ballet *Serenade*, provide a fun and effective mixture of classical ballet with fitness. Mat work like bridge exercises and *arabesque* extensions, along with *attitude* circles on one knee, target and tone the backside, shaping a dancer's form. Standing exercises such as *attitude* lifts, *grands pliés*, and even a basic *port de bras* front and back in the center further engage the glutes.

Piqué turn *sur le cou-de-pied*.

Piqué, meaning "pricked," is a sharp, bright step onto a straight standing knee with the working leg in *passé*, *attitude*, arabesque, or sur le *cou-de-pied* (pictured). *Piqués* are often performed in a series of turns traveling across the floor.

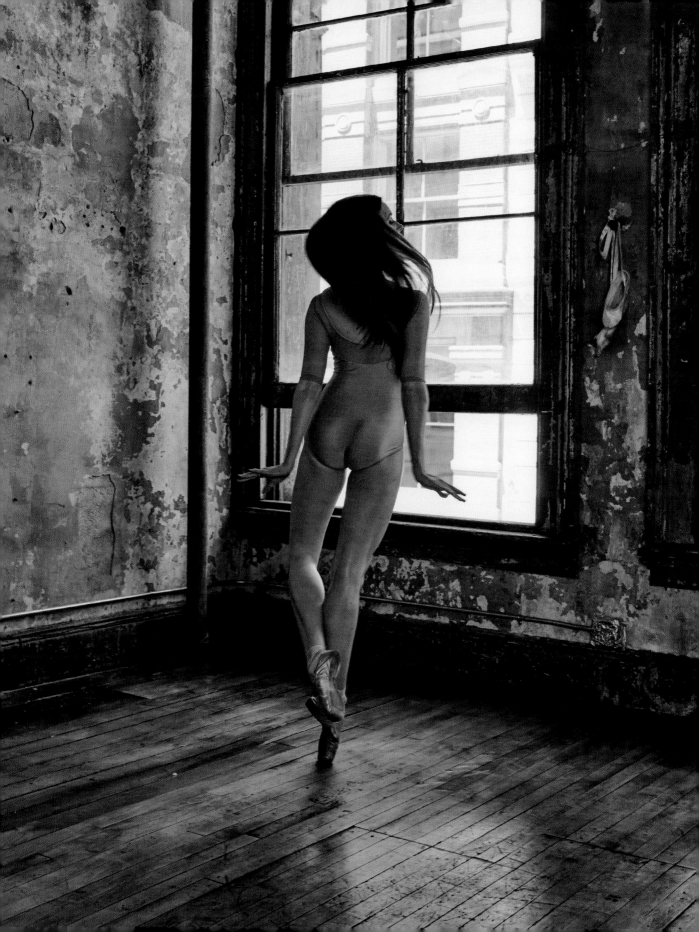

An *arabesque* on the stomach tones the muscles in the derrière, legs, and abs.

Dance Principle
Modified barre exercises like this *tendu* battement in arabesque build strength and muscle tone in the back of the thighs and derrière.

Fitness Tip
Lying on the stomach, bend one knee and extend the other leg into an arabesque. Pull in tight with the belly to balance and engage with the abs. Hold for one set of eight counts, then lift slightly higher and hold for another eight counts. Stretch and change sides. For more stability lower the bottom leg straight along the floor.

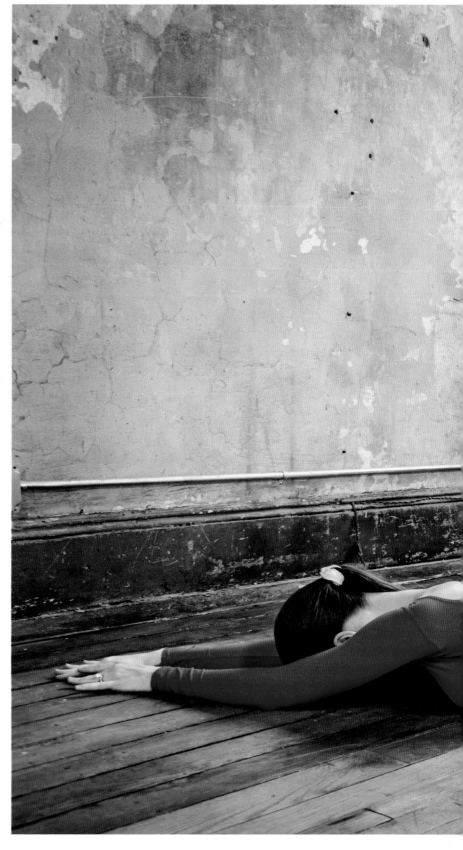

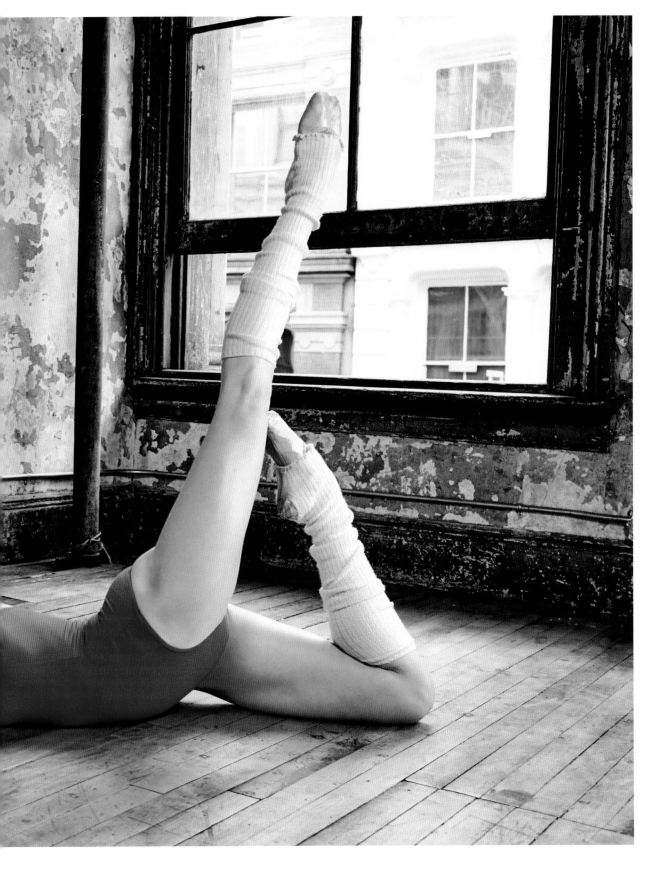

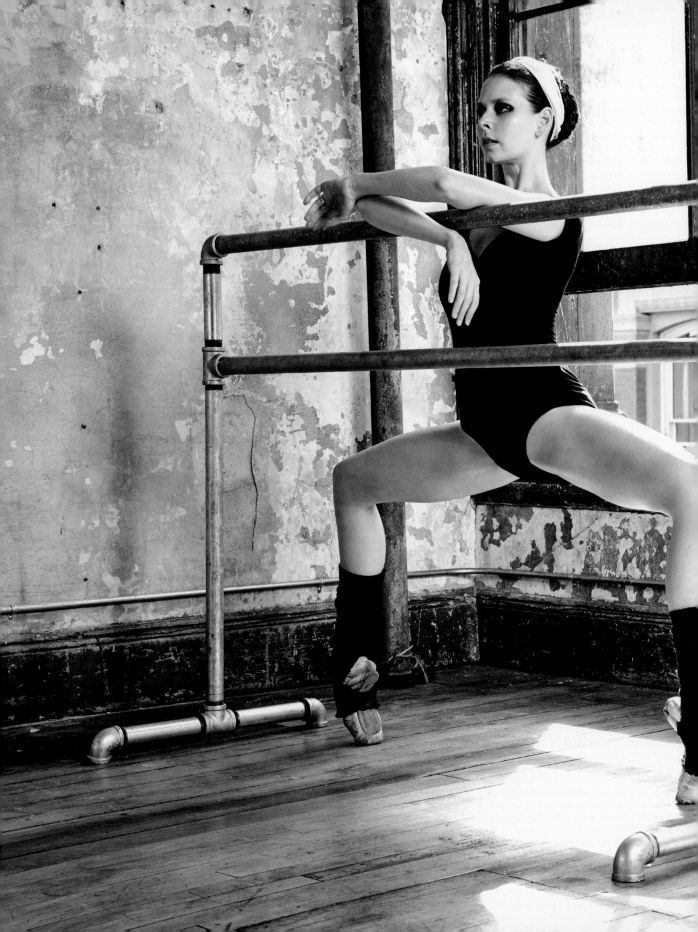

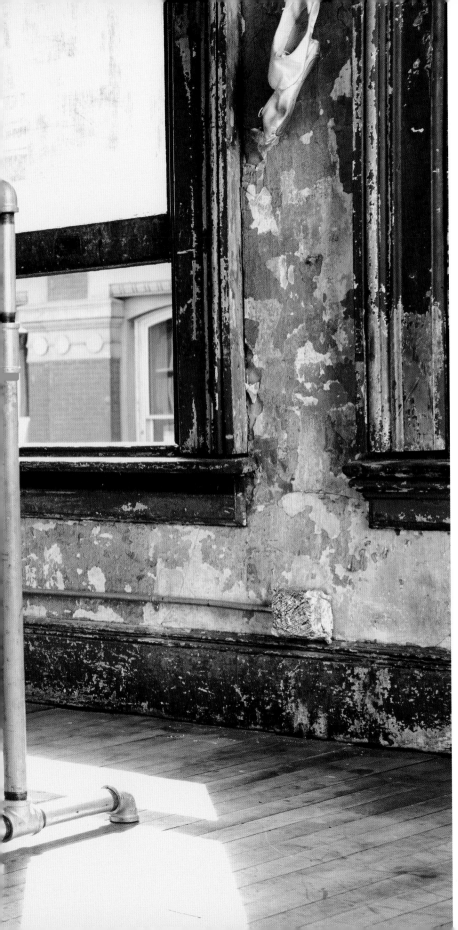

Grand *plié en pointe à la seconde*. *Plié* means "bent," and grand means "large," thus a grand *plié* is a deep bend of the knees. Practicing *en pointe* makes the movement more challenging, further engaging the muscles in the legs, *derrière*, and core.

Dance Principle
Keep the knees over the toes to protect the joints from over rotating and ensure that you are working within your range of motion. Pull the abs in tight to prevent any arch in the back.

Fitness Tip
No *pointe shoe*s? No problem! *Plié*s can be done with the feet flat, on *demi-pointe* (half pointe), or even in sneakers with fantastic results. Transform a squat into a grand *plié* in your next workout by simply turning the toes out—keeping the knees over the toes moves the tension from the quads to the inner thighs, core, and *derrière*.

91

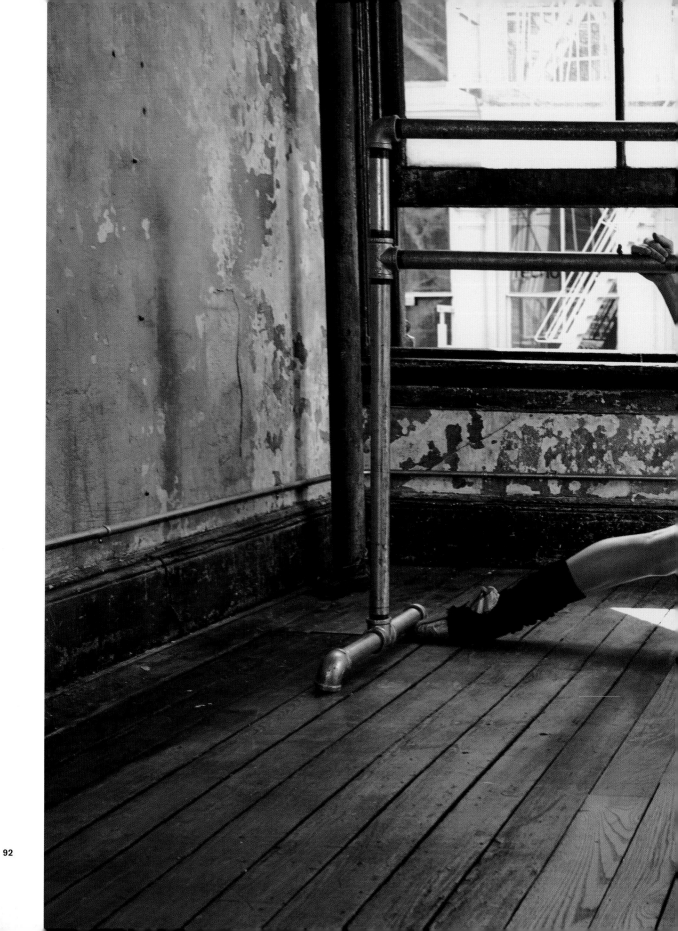

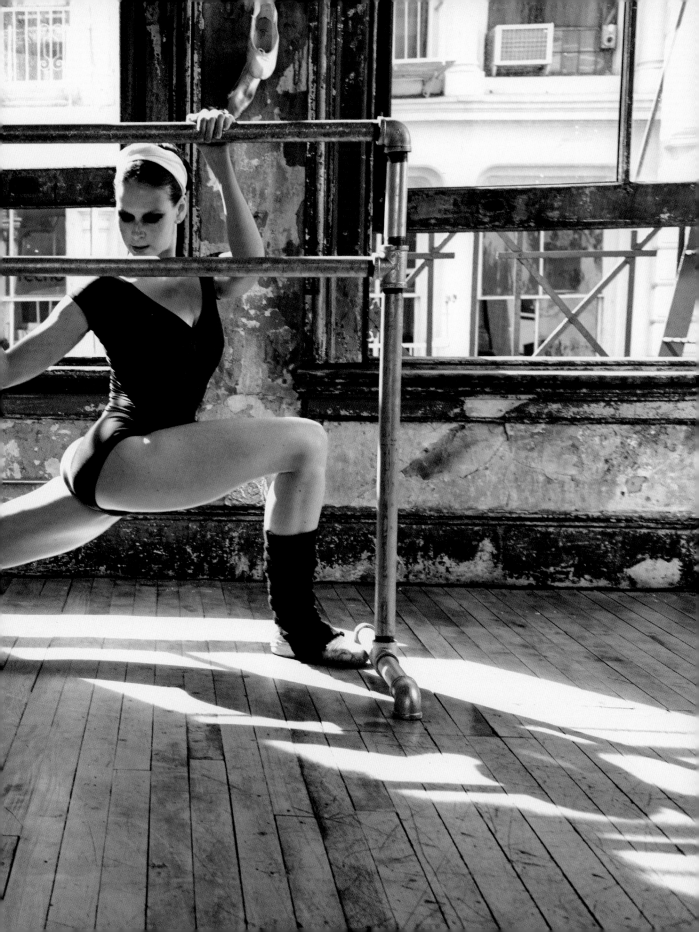

[PREVIOUS PAGES] A deep lunge at the barre opens the front of the hips while toning the derrière. If you don't have a ballet barre handy try using a wall, countertop, or chair for support.

Dance Principle
Stretching the fronts of the hips and thighs releases tension and lengthens the lines of the legs.

Pro Tip
Try releasing the hands from the barre at the bottom of this stretch to challenge your center of balance and achieve a serious, sculpting burn!

Fitness Tip
Once the muscles are warm, add this stretch in for a deep release. Lower and hold for two sets of eight, and then change sides.

[THIS PAGE + OPPOSITE] *Attitude* lifts at the barre lift and tone the derrière.

Dance Principle
Turning the hip inward changes the muscles targeted in a classic *attitude* back, engaging the muscles directly at the top of the hamstring and the back of the gluteus, where the thigh connects to the derrière.

Fitness Tip
Add a *plié* to your standing knee to make these *attitude* lifts work double duty, toning and sculpting the muscles on both the standing, working leg, and derrière. Beginning with the feet in sixth position (toes together, heels together), bend both knees and lift one leg into an *attitude* back with the hips in parallel. Keep the standing knee bent, pull the abs in tight, and bring the working foot toward the derrière with a light bounce. Hold and repeat for two to three sets of eight counts. Stretch and change sides.

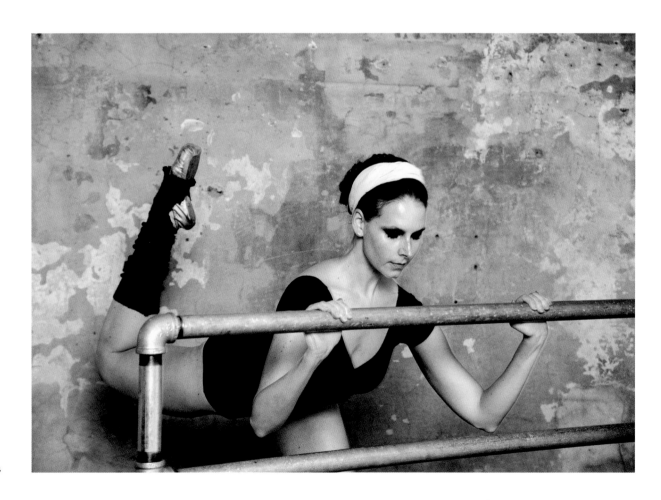

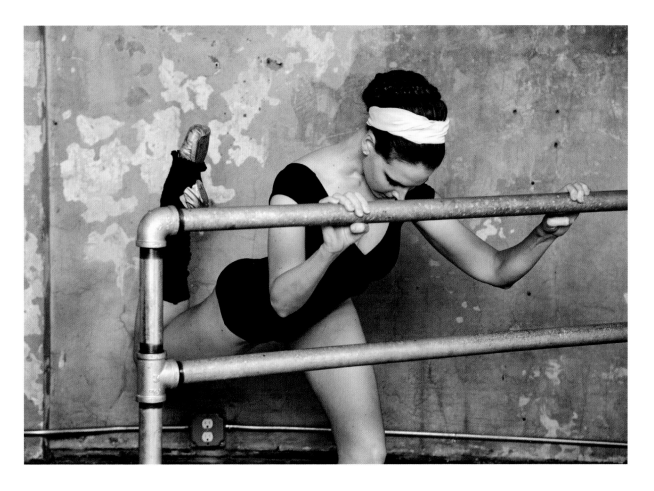

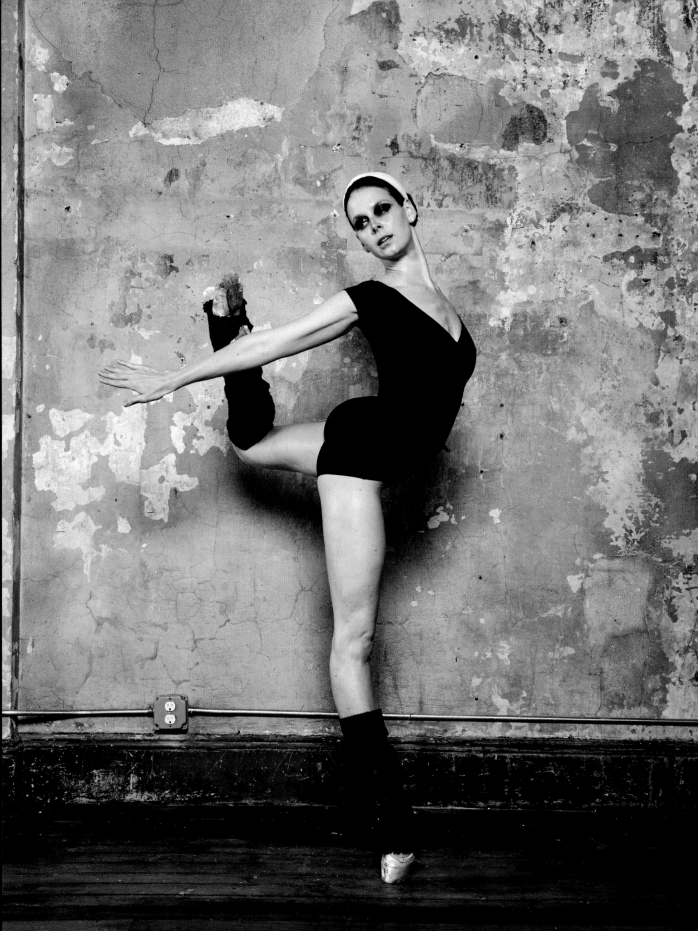

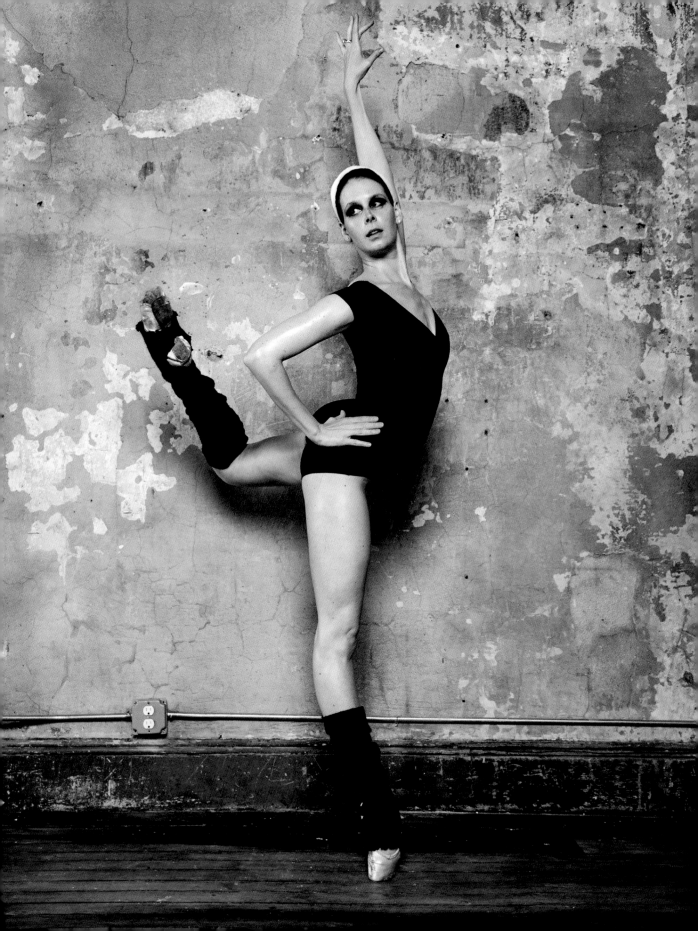

Dance Principle

A *pique attitude* lengthens the muscles in the standing leg while continuing to engage and strengthen the derriere. A twist through the waist engages the abdominals and obliques.

Fitness Tip

Try this exercise first at the barre for extra support. As you gain confidence and control through your center of balance, step away from the barre and practice in the center with the hands free. Begin with four to eight reps on each side. Step onto a straight knee with the abs pulled in tight, bending the back knee into an *attitude* position with the hip open and the back knee lifted. Begin the first set with both arms low. Stretch, change sides and repeat the set again this time lifting the same arm as working leg straight up while placing the other hand either on the barre or hip.

[THIS PAGE + OPPOSITE] *Attitude* leaps use every muscle in the body.

Dance Principle

Changing the arms and orientation of the front foot adds stylistic variation to *attitude* leaps. When jumping in the air, bend the front knee and lift the back thigh into an *attitude* with the knee bent into an *attitude* position.

Fitness Tip

No matter how high you go, these jumps make for a serious burn. *Plié* and leap up into the air, bending both knees, one to four times. Change sides and repeat.

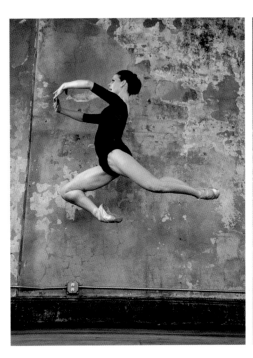

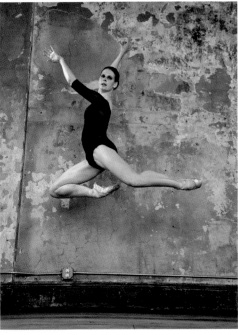

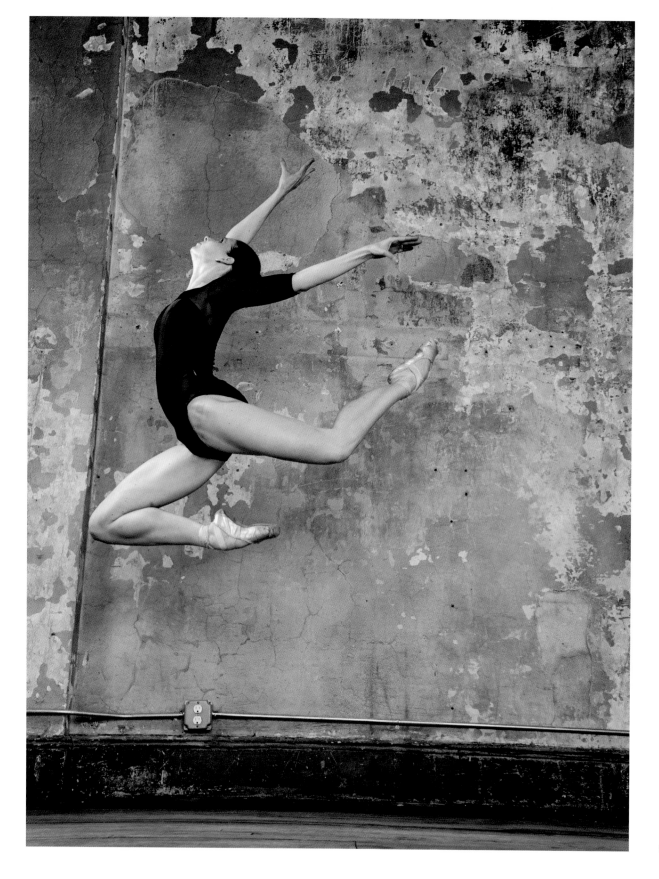

Lunge in *arabesque*

Dance Principle
A turned-out toe transforms a basic lunge into an *arabesque*, toning and targeting the thighs and *derrière*.

Fitness Tip
After your next cardio workout, add in a series of *arabesque* lunges to lift the *derrière* and sculpt sleek ballerina muscles. Begin with the feet together in sixth position (toes together, heels together). Spring forward into a lunge in *arabesque* with the arms open. Hop back to sixth position and repeat with the other leg in front for two sets of eight.

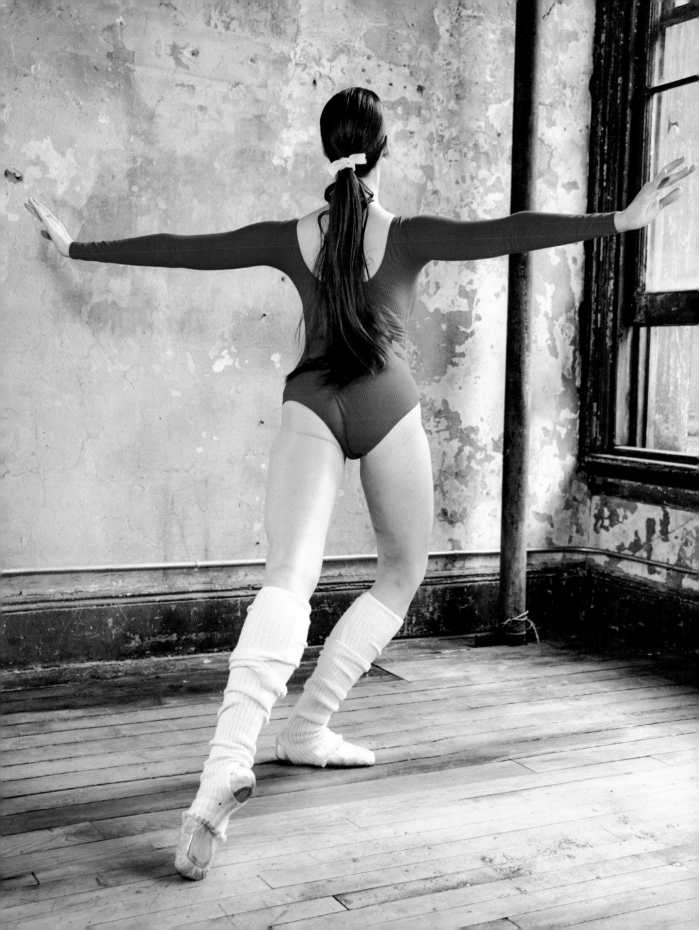

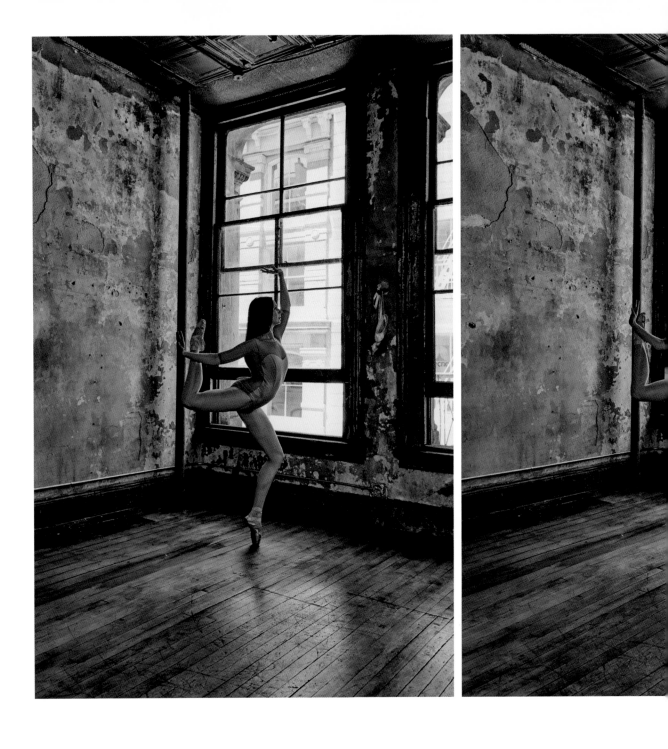

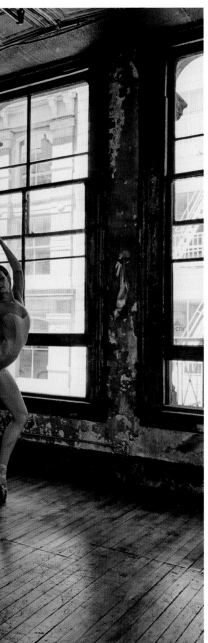

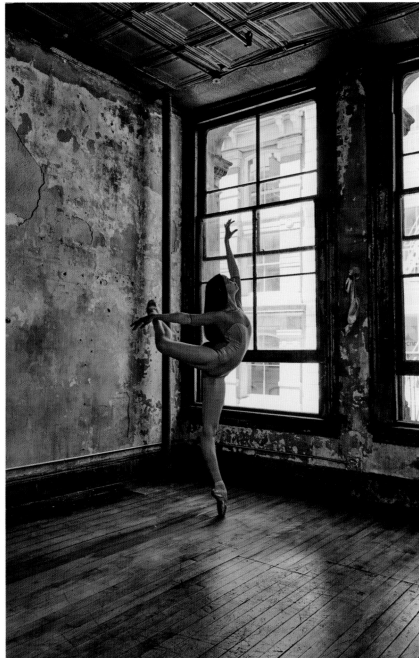

Piqué attitude en pointe.

Dance Principle
Whether the standing knee is bent or straight, and the hips turned out or in, the many variations of piqué *attitude*s provide great toning for the legs and derrière.

Pro Tip
Lift the back leg from the thigh and toe for higher extension and a more dramatic line.

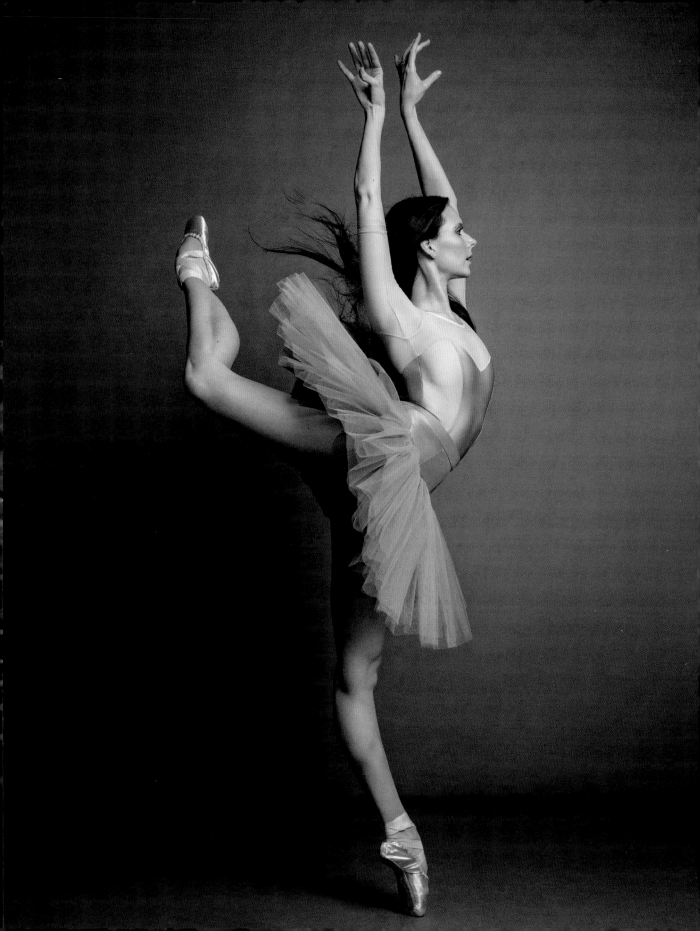

Posture

One of my favorite things about good posture is how contagious it is! Great posture helps us to better connect with our core and projects power and confidence at every age. Simply seeing someone in an upright and lifted position inspires you to do the same. Many a time I've sat down in a meeting to be told that just seeing me was a reminder to sit up straighter. If only all good habits were as easy to impart!

A ballerina is immediately recognizable for her elegant posture and beautiful carriage. Much like working and engaging the abdominals throughout each exercise, with ballet almost every position is executed with perfect posture, ingraining the habit into a dancer's muscle memory and physical form. Ballet Beautiful mirrors this process, incorporating an upright carriage and elegant posture into seemingly nonrelated exercises for the legs, butt, and core to build strength and solidify the habit.

One of the things that I love most about posture is that you can work on it anytime, anywhere, from sitting on your couch in your pj's to working at your desk or in a meeting, and even while grocery shopping—no leotard or ballet slippers required! The first step is getting into a good base position. The stomach is pulled in, tight and engaged, with the ribs closed (envision a zipper connecting the top of the ribcage) to prevent any arch in the back. Imagine someone pushing down ever so slightly on your shoulders while pulling the chest open from the middle of the back. Shoulders are open and the shoulder blades are pulled back and down. The neck is long with the chin relaxed but lifted.

This starting position provides the ideal foundation for building and maintaining great posture, bringing each of us closer to our inner Odette. Once this elemental position is achieved, we can strengthen and tone the arms with a mixture of light weights, no weights, and high reps. When it comes to working on posture, I always remind my clients to think like a swan.

Sous-sus with *cambré* back.

Dance Principle
Beautiful posture is an integral part of ballet training, resulting from a combination of flexibility and strength in the upper body.

Pro Tip
Imagine a drop of water running from your shoulders down to your fingertips as you lift up and open through the chest.

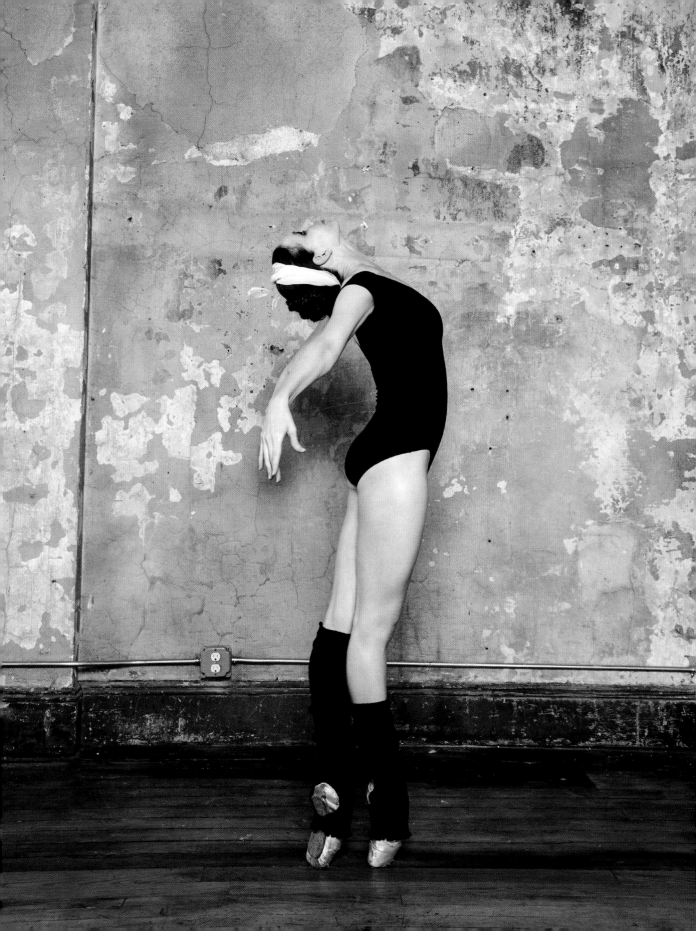

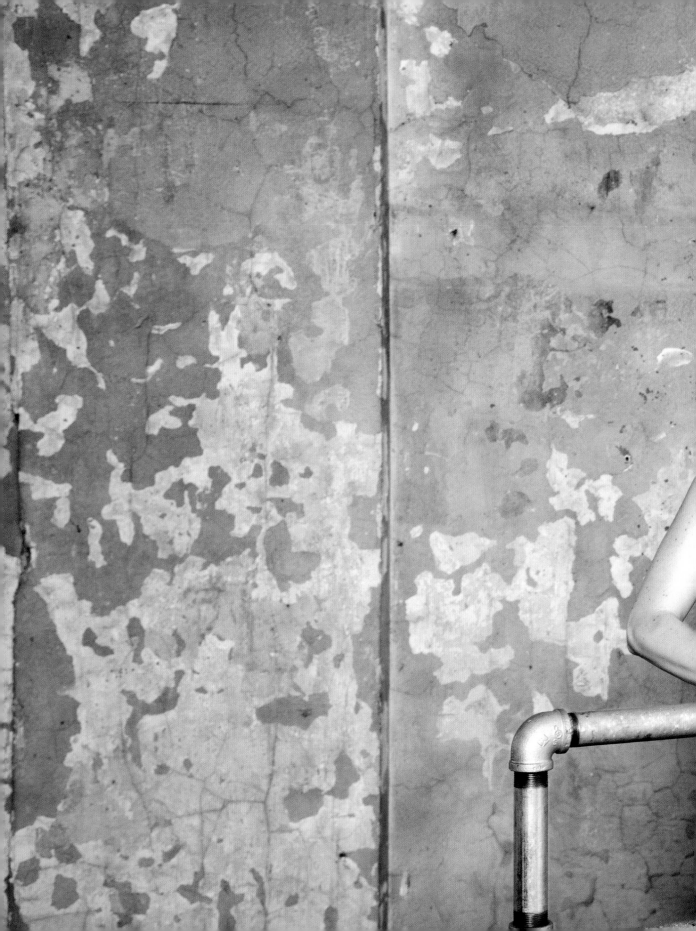

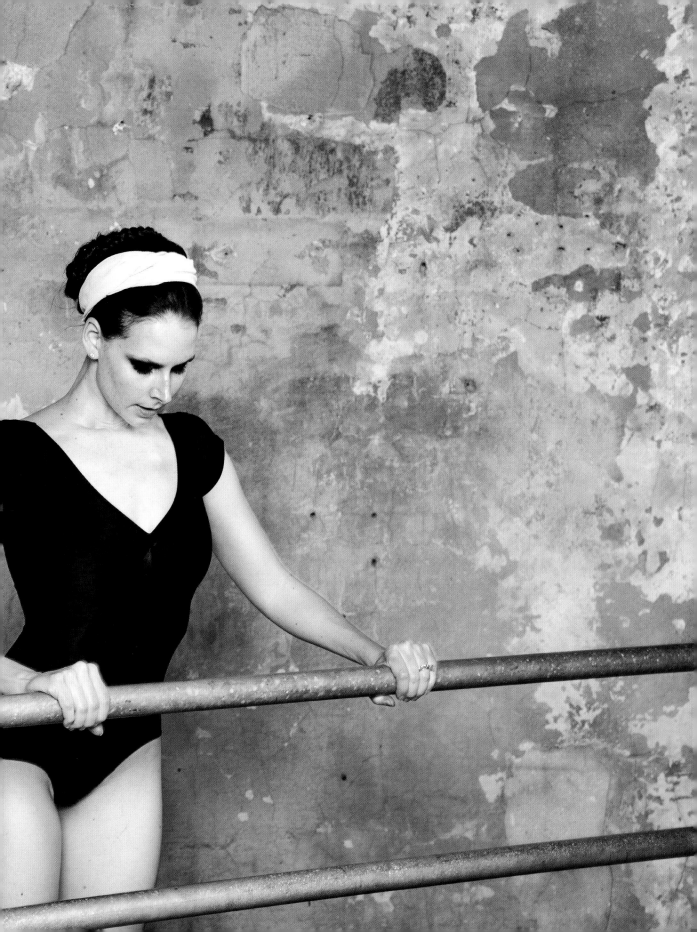

[PREVIOUS PAGES]

Dance Principle
For dancers, great posture begins at the barre. Simple stretches and exercises build strength and awareness through the back and core.

Fitness Tip
A ballet barre is a terrific tool for stretching and opening the chest and upper body. If you are training from home or outside of a dance studio, try using a countertop or windowsill that is thigh or hip height while being sturdy enough to bear weight. Place the hands shoulder-width apart, pushing down through the shoulders to lengthen the neck while opening through the back and chest. Pull the stomach in tight and press the elbows down. Hold for sixteen counts.

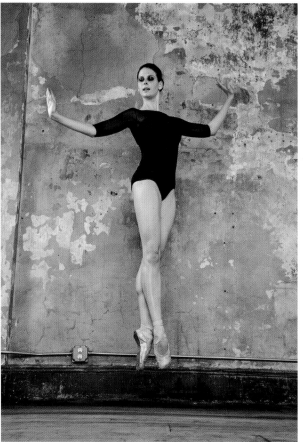

Allegro: [THIS PAGE] Soubresaut. [OPPOSITE] *Assemblé* en avant.

A soubresaut is a jump straight into the air where the legs are held straight and the feet cross in fifth position in the air. Allegro means "happy." As a dance term, it is applied to brisk, energetic jumps in the center of the room, ranging from small (petit) to large (grand) movements. *Assemblé* means "joined together" or "assembled." In an *assemblé* en avant (front) the legs brush forward off the ground, closing together into fifth position in the air.

Dance Principle
Pushing down through the shoulders and opening the chest stabilizes the upper body while jumping.

Fitness Tip
Ballet-inspired jumps provide great cardio while building beautiful posture. Open the arms out to the side into second position. Open the chest and pull the abs in tight as you jump, stretching both knees long and crossing the ankles in the air. Repeat this jump four to eight times, and then stretch and change sides.

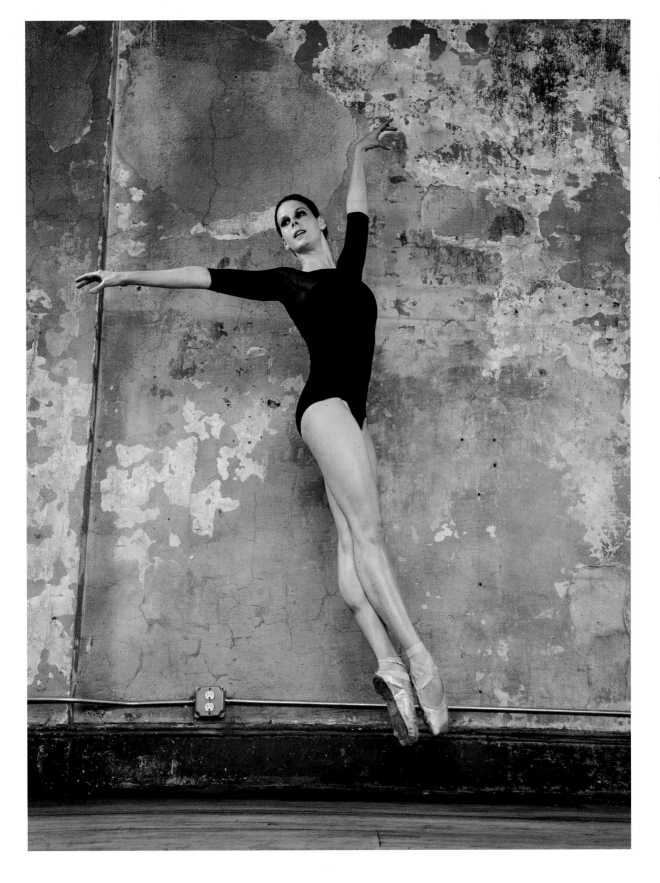

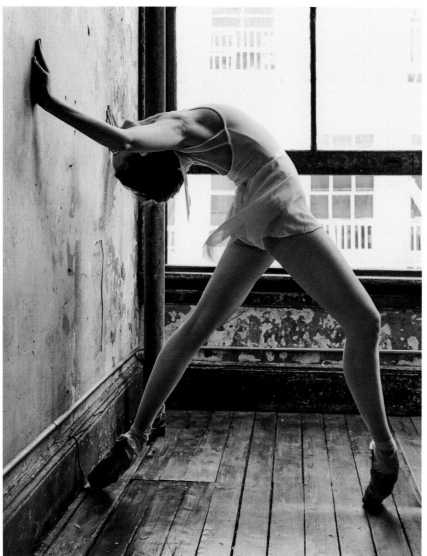

Cambré derrière en pointe.

Dance Principle
Flexibility and strength play equally
important roles in achieving elegant
posture. Back bends, or *cambré*s *en
pointe* build control through the back
and core and open up the upper body.

Fitness Tip
A modified version of this movement
is a great way to incorporate ballerina
posture in your next workout. Begin
with the legs in fourth position, one
foot in front of the other, bending the
front leg. Place the hands on the hips,
pull in with the abdominals, and lift
both arms up and over the head, with a
slight arch in the back. Slowly lift the
upper body back to an upright position,
lower the arms, and change sides.

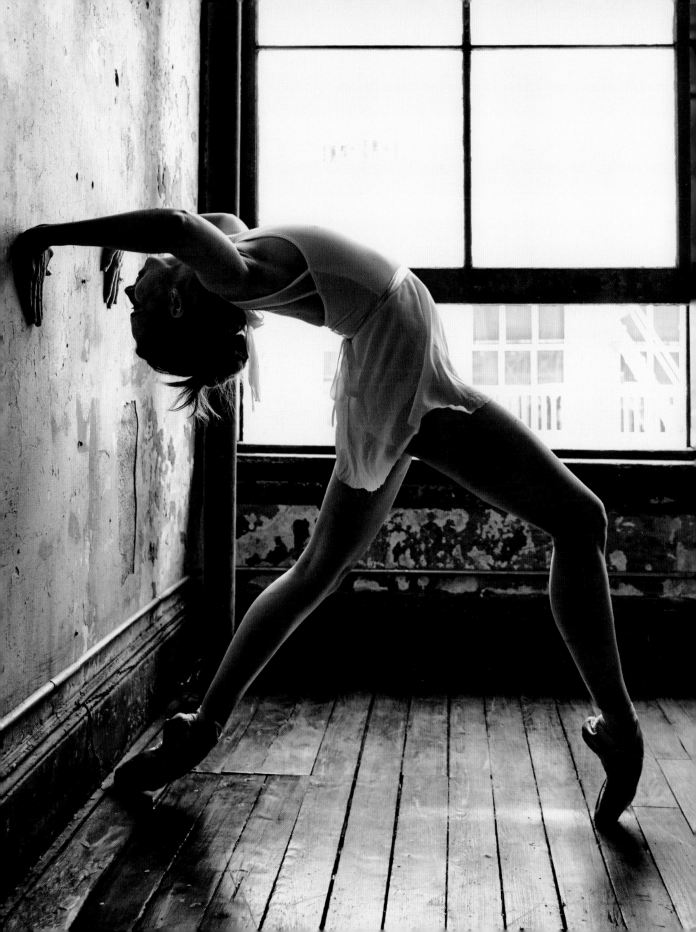

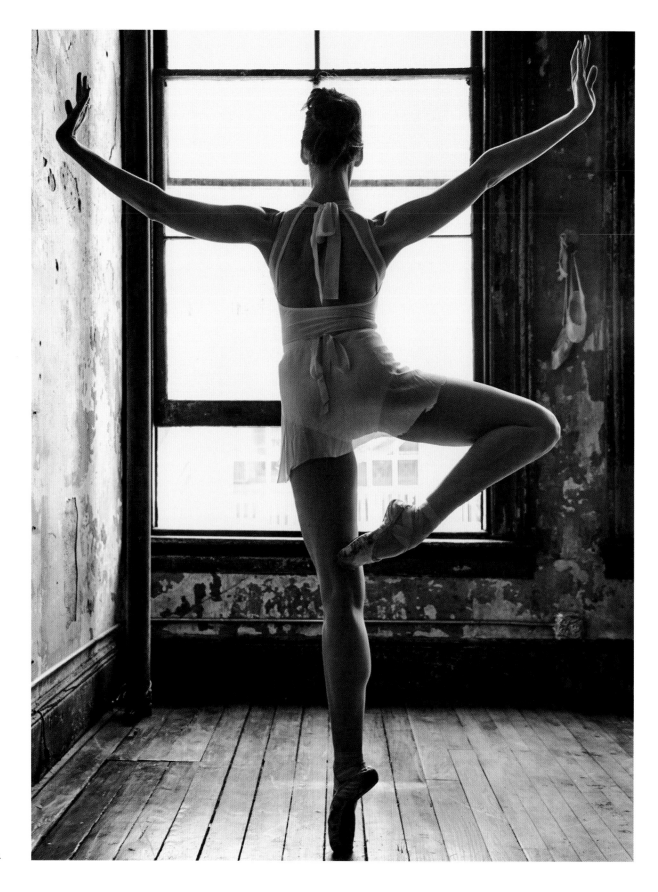

[OPPOSITE] *Piqué passe* with arms to the side.

Dance Principle

Pushing the arms open and to the sides strengthens the back while engaging the core.

Fitness Tip

Lift the hands to the ears and stretch the elbows long, pushing down through the shoulders as you open the chest. Set your timer and hold for two minutes.

[THIS PAGE] *Tendu plié en avant.*

Dance Principle

This simple *tendu plié* works the legs, core, arms and back. Imagine one long line between the front toe in *tendu* and the back arm, lifting up and stretching long behind you.

Fitness Tip

Find the opposition in your back as you take a *tendu* front, bending the standing knee. Stretch the same arm as working leg up and back, twisting through the upper body. Reach down towards the toe in *tendu* with the opposite elbow while continuing to extend the back arm long behind you. Engage the core and open the chest up and slightly back, taking care to stay lifted and not collapse through the upper body.

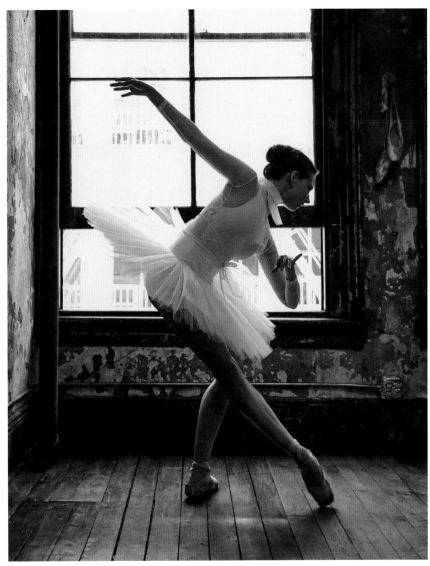

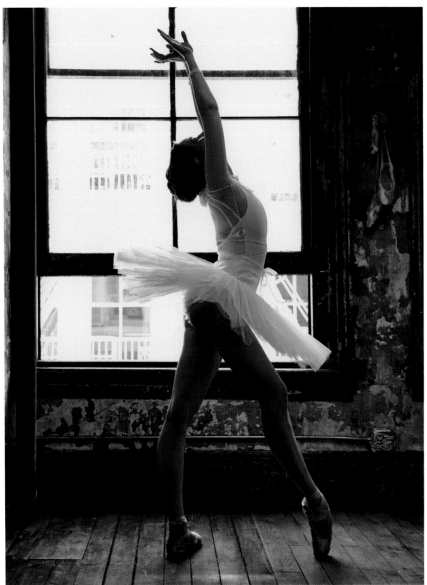

[THIS PAGE + OPPOSITE] *Port de bras*, meaning "carriage of the arms," builds strength and muscle tone to maintain elegant ballerina posture.

Dance Principle
The push and pull between lifting up with the arms and pressing down through the shoulders adds resistance and challenge to a basic *port de bras*.

Dance Principle
Swan arms come in many variations. This *port de bras* with the wrists across the forehead and hips is reminiscent of Swan Lake.

Fitness Tip
Make swan arms a part of your workout! Open and stretch the arms to the side into second position, engaging the abs and opening through the chest. Cross the arms, bringing the top wrist to the forehead and the opposite wrist to the center of the ribs. Stretch arms back to second position and change sides. Repeat for four sets of eight, alternating sides each time.

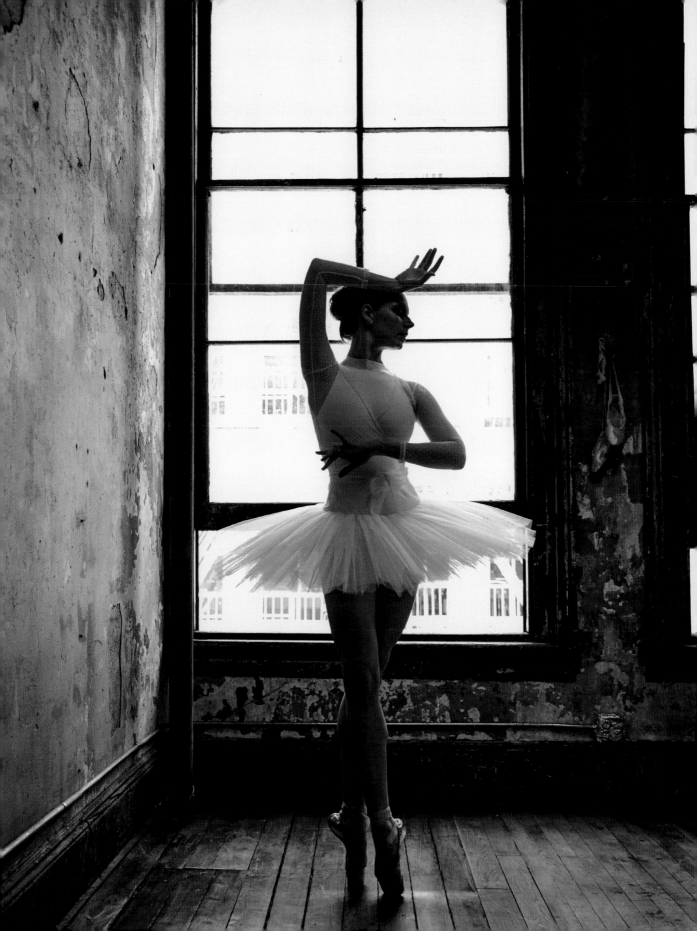

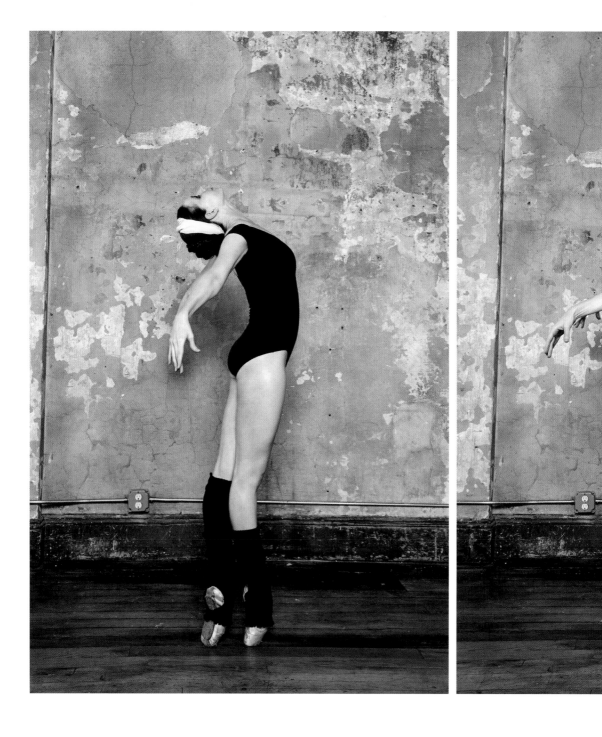

Sous-sus series with *cambré derrière*. *Sous-sus* means "over, under" while *cambré* means "arched." Here we see the feet pulled together and crossed at the ankles in a *relevé* in fifth position, with the arms and upper body arching up and back.

Dance Principle
Great posture originates in the upper back.

Pro Tip
Imagine a figurehead at the bow of a ship arching forward into the seas as you lift the arms and stretch through the back.

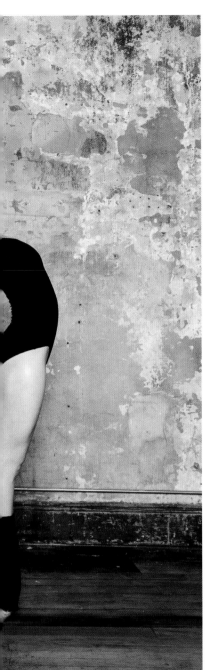
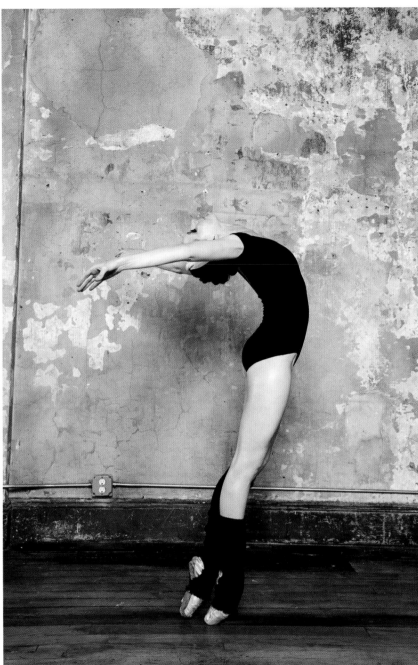

Fitness Tip
Start by practicing this movement with the feet flat. As you build strength and confidence, the heels may be lifted onto a *demi-pointe* for greater challenge. Begin by lining the front heel up to the back toe in third position, bend the knees into a *plié* and lift the arms up and back as you stretch both knees. Repeat three times, and then change sides.

Cool down stretch in *passé* parallel.

Dance Principle
The opposition and resistance between the working leg and spine releases tension and tightness in the back and upper body after a challenging class, workout, or performance.

Pro Tip
Let your breath help you deepen your stretch and release tension. Take a deep breath in and slowly exhale as your body twists into this *passé* stretch.

Fitness Tip
This stretch is most effective post workout, when the muscles are already warm. Begin lying on the mat and bend one knee and lift to the chest, keeping the hip turned in. Lift the opposite arm up and above the head. Roll the working (bent) knee toward the opposite leg, dropping the knee on the floor as you twist through the spine and waist looking away. Release the breath and hold for two sets of eight, and then change sides.

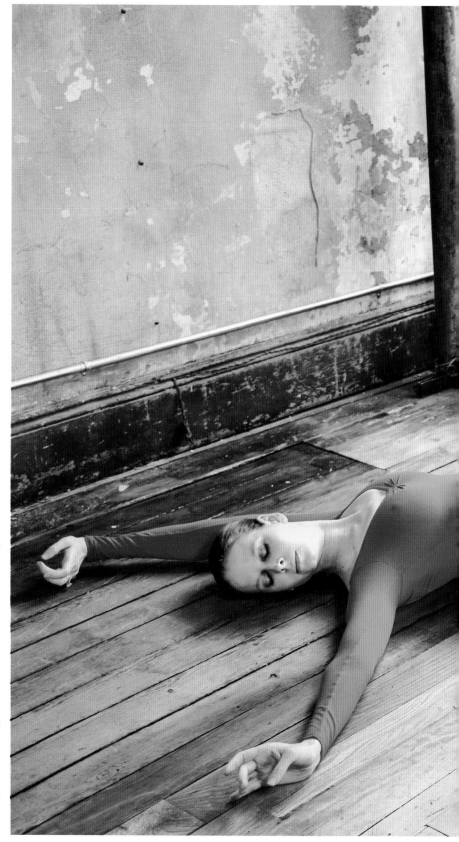

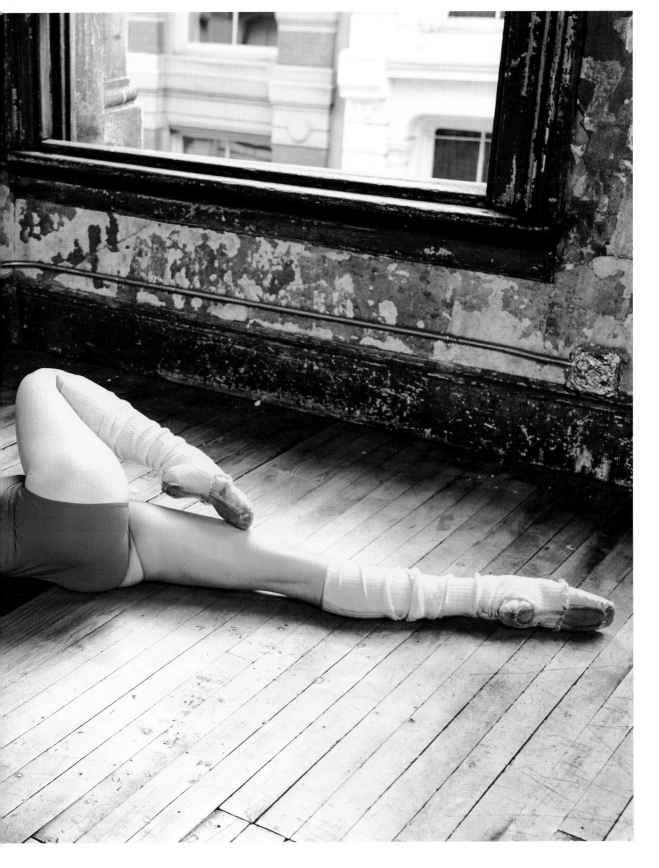

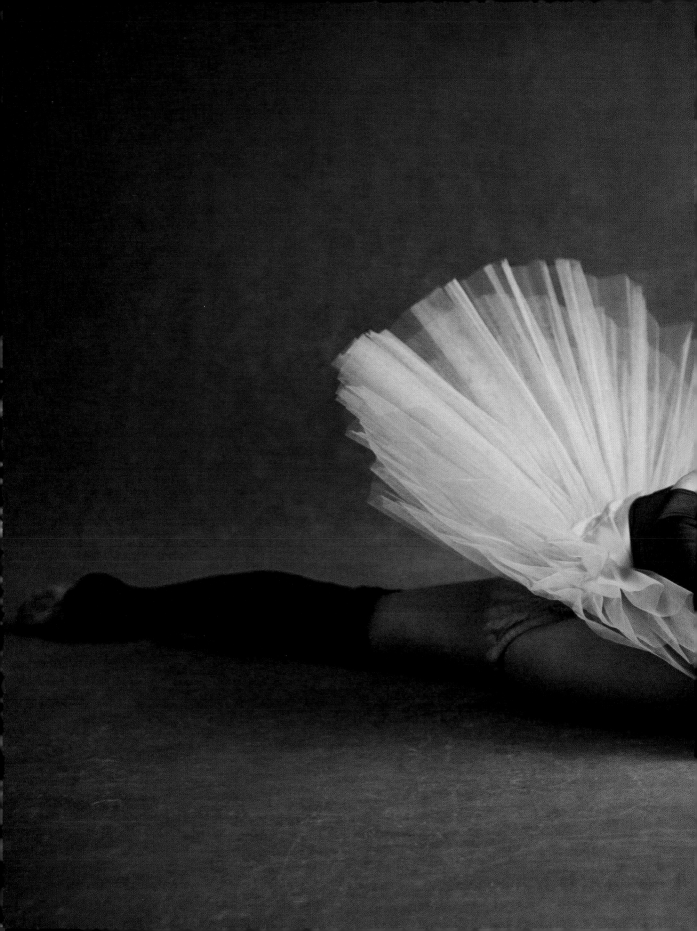

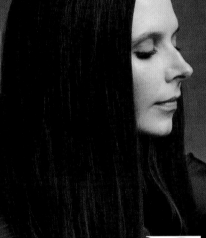

1.6

Flexibility

Dancers stretch all day long. Lengthening, moving, and extending through the limbs and muscles is as natural as breathing for a ballerina. Stretching elongates muscles, relieves tension, and increases flexibility, helping to lengthen a dancer's line. An essential part of classical ballet, stretching is incorporated before, after, and during every class, rehearsal, performance, and, by extension, every Ballet Beautiful workout.

Consistency is key to increasing flexibility. Whether trying to achieve a full split, increase agility, or simply touch your toes, all of us can become more flexible over time with daily stretching. When I was a young girl dreaming of moving to New York City to become a ballerina I would lie in bed at night thinking about how I could make it happen. I would close my eyes and make to-do lists of how I could work harder to improve my technique and become more flexible like the professional ballerinas I so admired. I spent my free time working on my splits to increase my extension and lift my legs higher in ballet class. I even trained myself to sleep in a frog position with the soles of my feet together and my hips open to improve my turnout. While sleeping in a split or frog is not a Ballet Beautiful requirement, (or even recommendation!) regular stretching works wonders for building and maintaining flexibility in everyday life.

When it comes to stretching it's important to remember that we are all put together a bit differently and so have a different range of motion. You may have noticed that one leg or side of your body is stronger or more agile than the other. The same is true for flexibility. I am much more open on my right side than on my left. I have better turnout, a higher *penché* (a ballet step that looks like a standing split with one foot on the ground and the other lifted high above, often in the "six o'clock" position) and a higher *arabesque* on my right side. While the difference is only a few degrees and in some cases might not even be noticeable to others, to me the contrast in flexibility between these two sides could not be more apparent! I have to carefully manage the desire to match my left side to my right in order not to push beyond my body's natural range of motion and overstretch or tax my joints. With stretching we must strike a balance between challenging and respecting the body's natural limits.

A simple standing hamstring stretch releases muscles in the back of the legs.

Pro Tip
Loose hamstrings help with splits, *grands jetés*, and hitting that six o'clock *penché* (a standing split in *arabesque* with one toe above the head and the other on the floor). For a deeper stretch, hold on to the ankles or shins, pulling the upper body as close to the thighs as possible while stretching the knees.

Fitness Tip
Incorporate this simple standing stretch before or after cardio and standing work to elongate the muscles in the legs. Bend forward and reach toward the ankles (or shins) while stretching the knees. Fold the upper body in half, pressing the upper body toward the thighs to increase the stretch. Hold for one to two sets of eight counts and slowly release the breath.

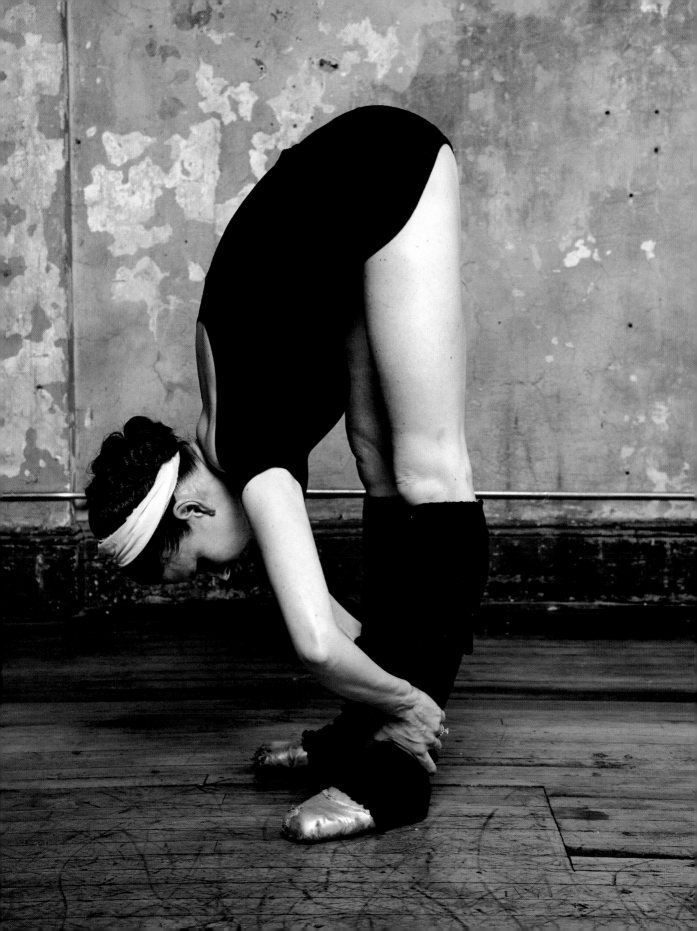

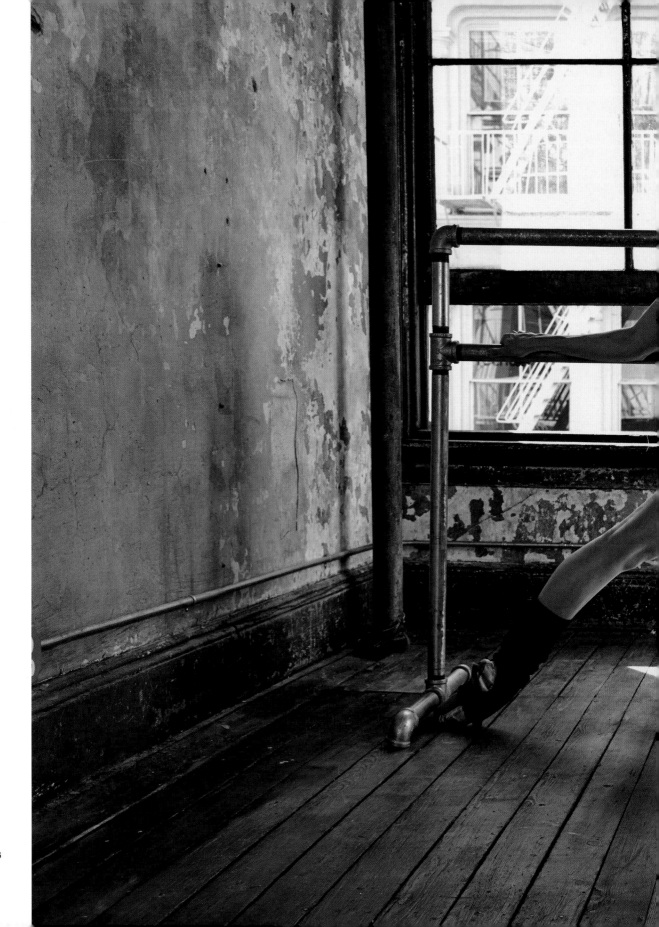

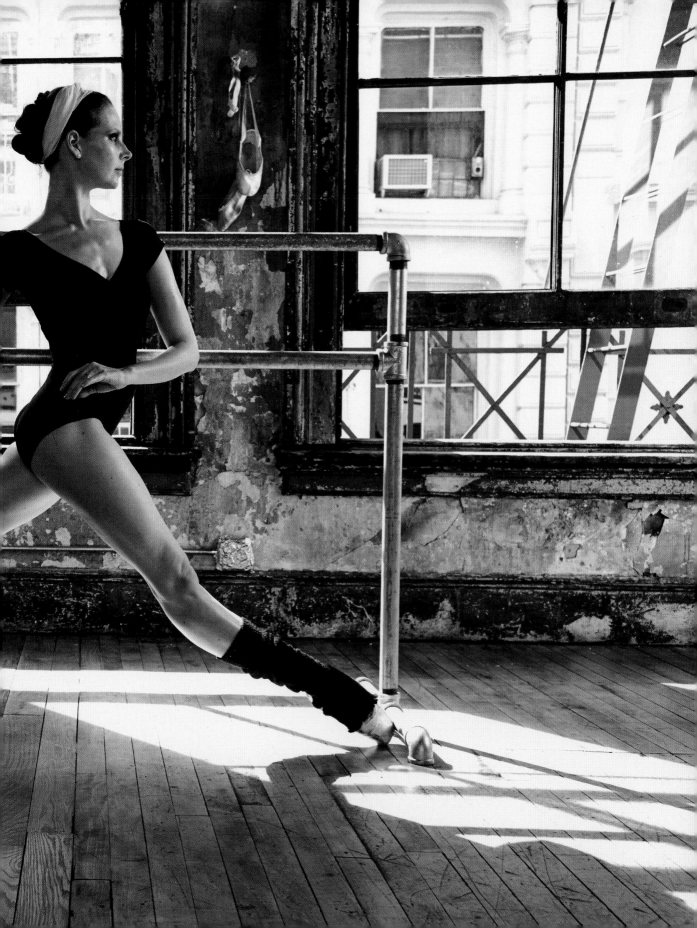

[PREVIOUS PAGES] Fourth position *en pointe*.

Dance Principle

A simple turn of the shoulders transforms a balance in fourth position into an upper body stretch and core workout.

Fitness Tip

Put a twist on it: stretching the body in more ways than one can make a workout more challenging—and effective. Open the legs into a wide fourth position, placing one foot in front of the other with the body balanced in between the legs. Pull in tight through the abs, and twist through the waist, turning to one side. Hold for one set of eight counts, then change sides.

[THIS PAGE + OPPOSITE] Classic hamstring stretches at the barre.

Dance Principle

The barre is the perfect place to start and finish a dancer's daily training. If you are working at home or backstage and don't have a barre handy, try finding a hard surface, such as a windowsill or a chair that is somewhere between mid-thigh to hip height (the higher the surface, the deeper the stretch). A classic hamstring stretch releases muscles and builds flexibility in the thighs legs, back, and hips. Using the weight of the body to roll muscles out along the barre releases tension and targets knots and other localized tight spots.

[THIS PAGE]
Fitness Tip

Lift one leg up to the front, placing the foot on a barre or sturdy surface. Bend forward and reach toward the toes while keeping both knees straight. Hold for three sets of eight counts, then change sides.

[THIS PAGE]
Pro Tip

Flex the foot to extend the stretch from the hamstring to the calf.

[OPPOSITE]
Pro Tip

Transform a barre stretch into a mini massage by using the body's weight to target tight muscles while rolling them out along the barre.

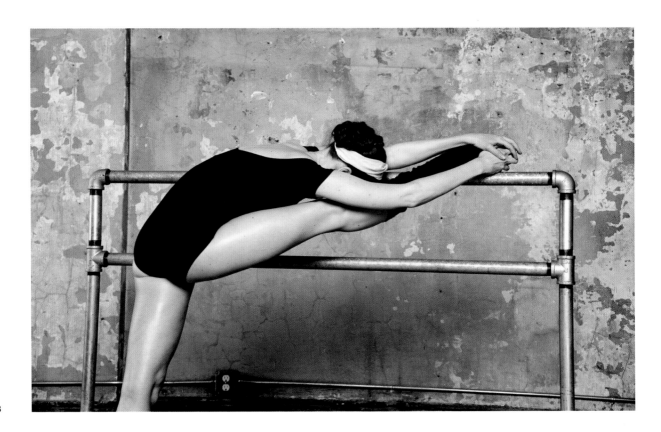

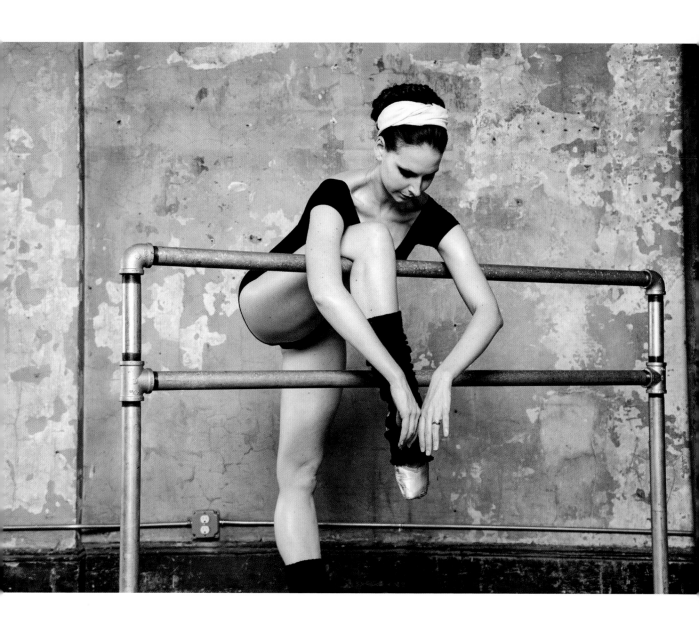

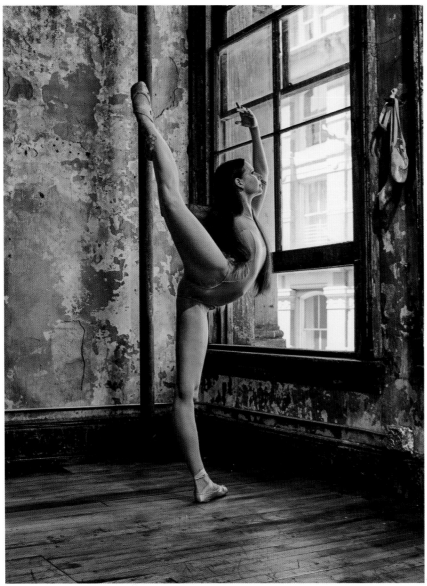

Standing *attitude* stretch.

Dance Principle
These standing stretches increase flexibility and range of motion in the back, for a higher *attitude* or *arabesque*.

Pro Tip
Lift the chest and upper body up and in as you pull the working foot toward the head for a deeper stretch.

Fitness Tip
Start where you are and work within your range of motion! A standing *attitude* stretch does not have to reach above your head. Begin by lifting the working leg back and bending the knee to ninety degrees. Place the hand opposite the working leg on the barre or wall for stability, and the hand on the same side as the working leg on the knee. Slowly lift the leg up in *attitude* while pulling in with the stomach and opening the chest.

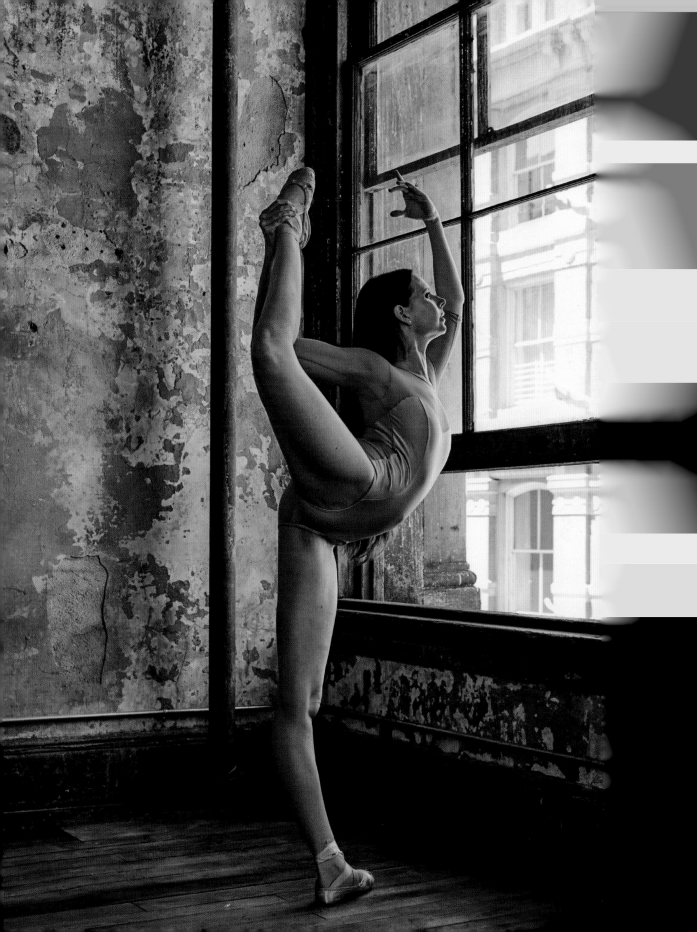

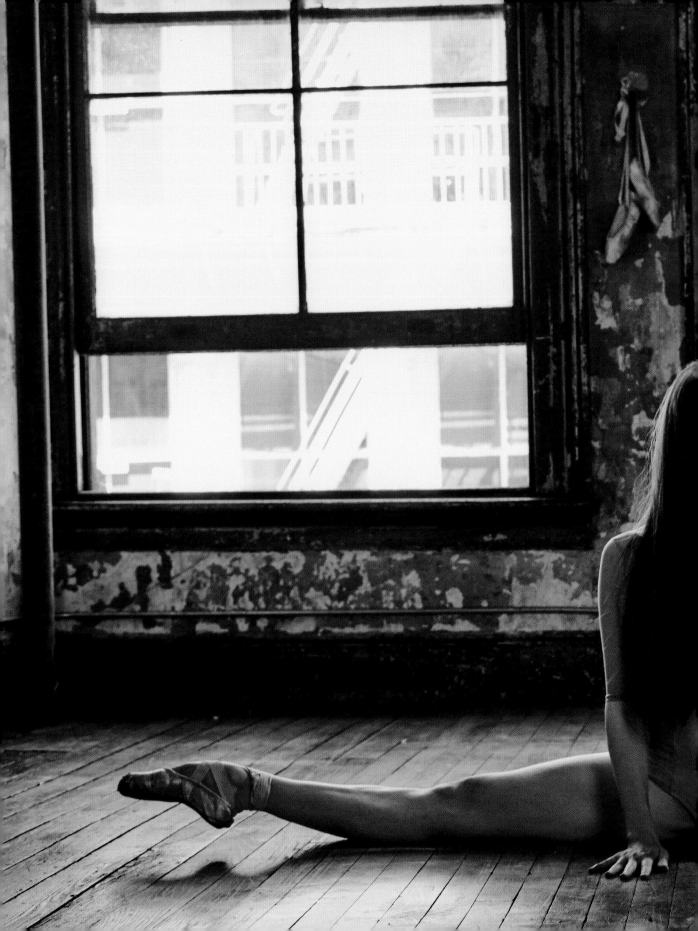

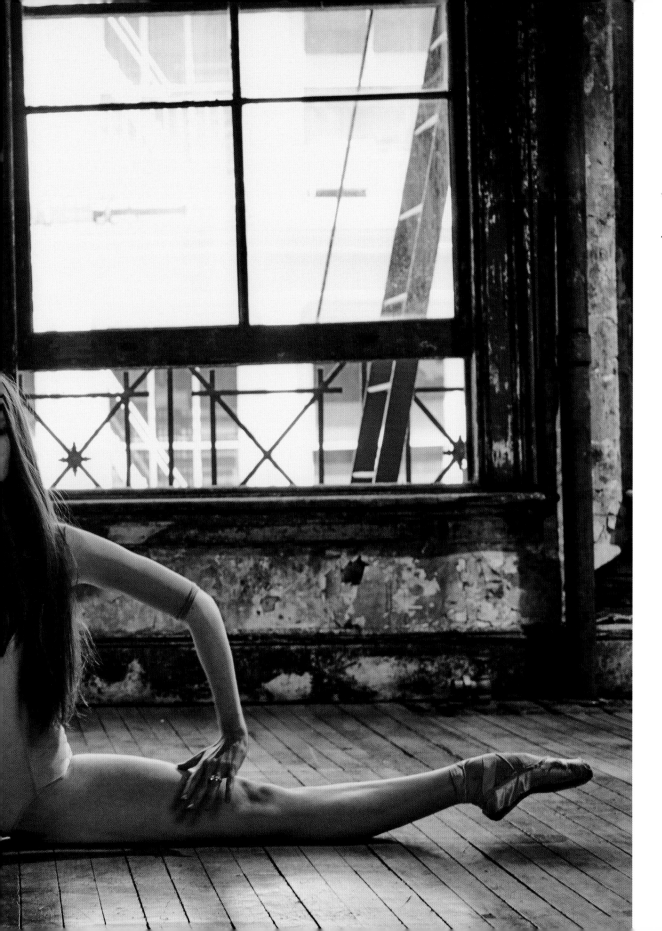

[PREVIOUS PAGES] Center splits play an important role in a dancer's daily training.

Pro Tip

Put your hands on the floor and push the hips forward to deepen the stretch and align the toes and hips.

[THIS PAGE + OPPOSITE] Center split with *port de bras* to the side and a forward bend.

Dance Principle

Upper body stretches add complexity and depth to a basic center split.

Pro Tip

Increase your range of motion through the hips and legs and release tension through the upper body with a *port de bras* to the side and a front bend lowering the upper body forward along the floor.

Fitness Tip

From a seated position, open the feet on the ground to a "Y" shape in front of you. Scoot the hips up and forward while pushing the feet open to the side and back toward the upper body, slowly working toward achieving a 180-degree angle with the legs and hips over time. Once you find the positioning for the legs and feet that feels best, add a *port de bras*! Lift one arm up and bend toward the opposite foot to deepen the stretch in the inner thighs and sides. Hold and repeat on the other side. For a deeper stretch, lift the body back to center and begin to move the hands forward on the floor into a forward bend, bringing the elbows down and dropping the head to release tension in the back, hips, legs, and upper body. For a deeper stretch, hold each position for two to four sets of eight.

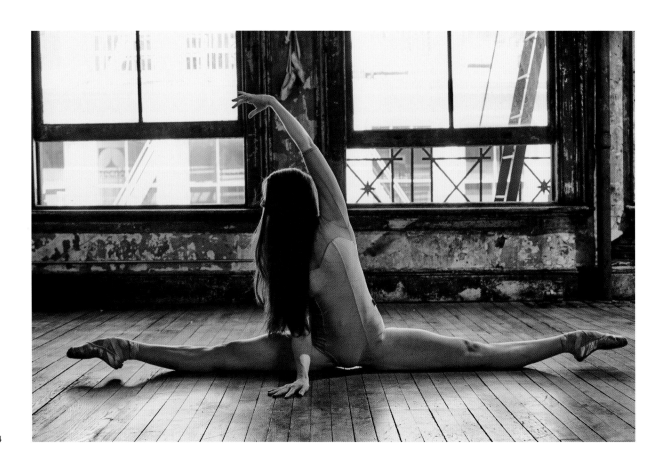

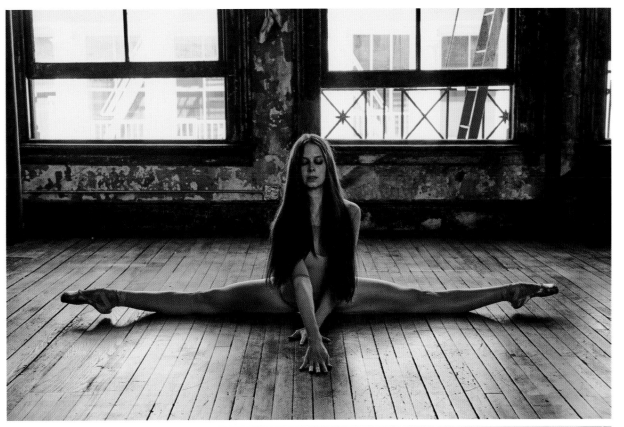

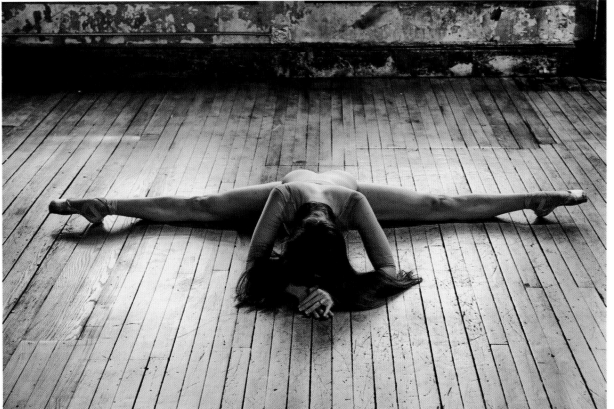

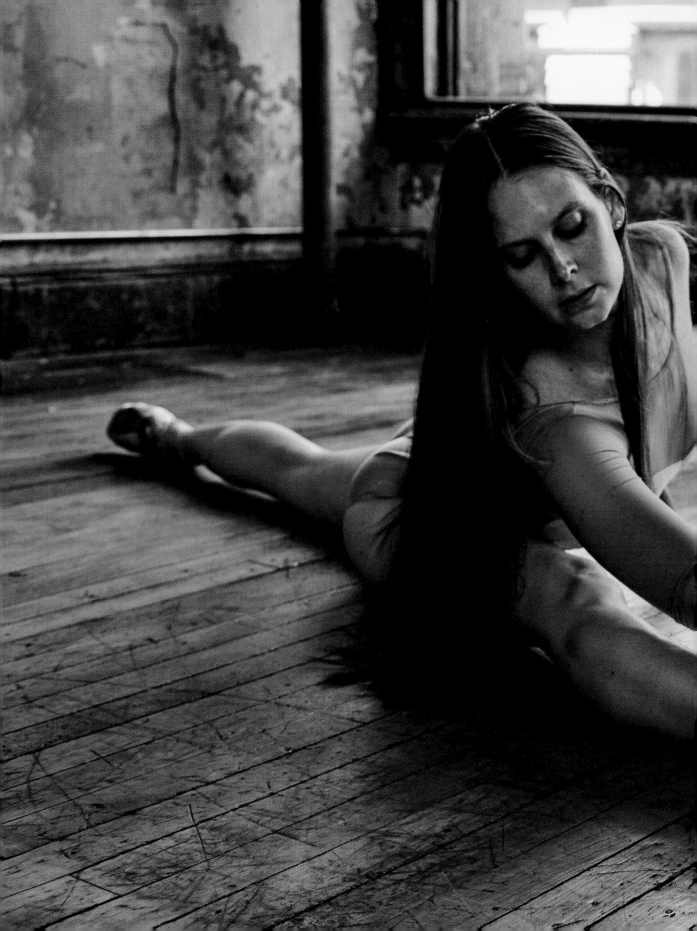

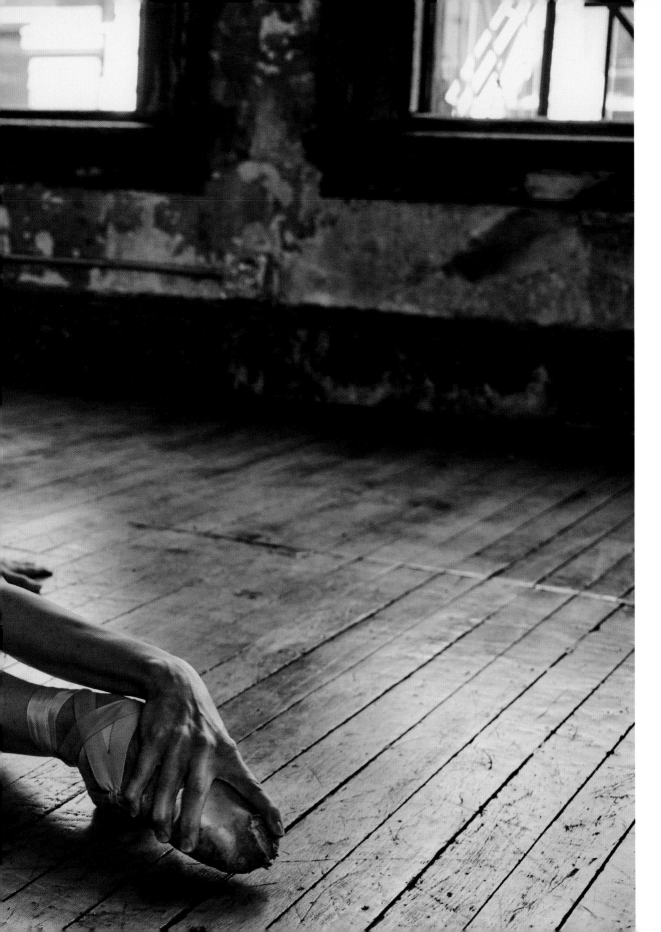

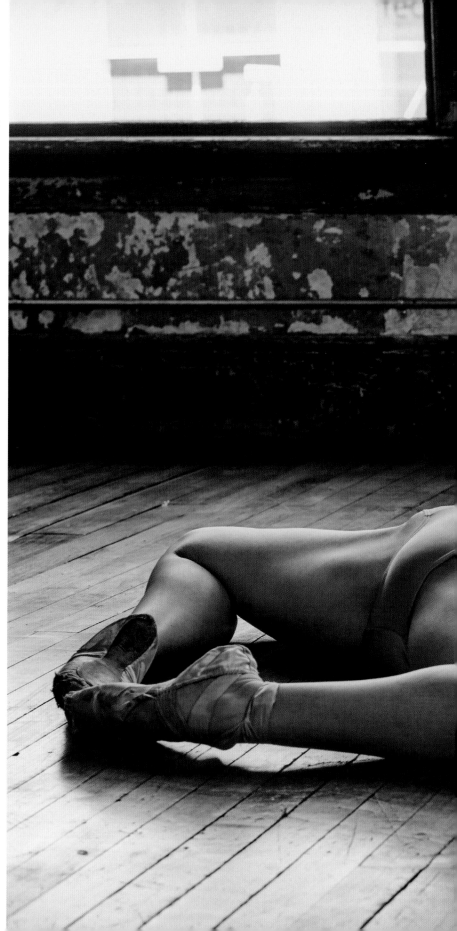

[PREVIOUS PAGES] Front split.

Dance Principle

A front split is a wonderful opener for the hips and legs that prepares the body for a larger range of movement including *grands jetés* (large leaps in the air), *développés*, and *grands battements* at the barre and in the center.

Pro Tip

Start slow and be patient! Flexibility is something that increases over time.

Fitness Tip

Use the hands to help guide your body into a deeper stretch. Extend one foot to the front and one to the back. Depending on your range of motion, your hips may be lifted off the floor. Place the hands on either side of the hips while working toward slowly stretching both knees and lowering the body into a split. Once you achieve your full range of motion, reach toward the front toe or shin with the same arm as leg to deepen the stretch through the legs and hips.

[OPPOSITE] Reclined "butterfly" stretch.

Dance Principle

"Turnout," or an openness of the hips, plays an important role in ballet technique. Butterfly stretches with the toes pulled together and the knees pushed down toward the floor can be performed seated or reclined to open the hips and increase turnout and range of motion.

Pro Tip

A classic butterfly stretch is performed sitting up. Performing this stretch lying down (pictured) increases pressure on the hips, making this fundamental ballet stretch more challenging and effective.

Fitness Tip

Add this simple hip opener to your warm-up and cooldown to release tension and increase openness through the hips. Begin by lying on the floor. Bring the toes together and open the legs, lowering the knees toward the floor. Place the arms above the head in fifth position and pull the belly in tight to engage the abs while allowing for a natural arch of the back. Hold for sixteen counts.

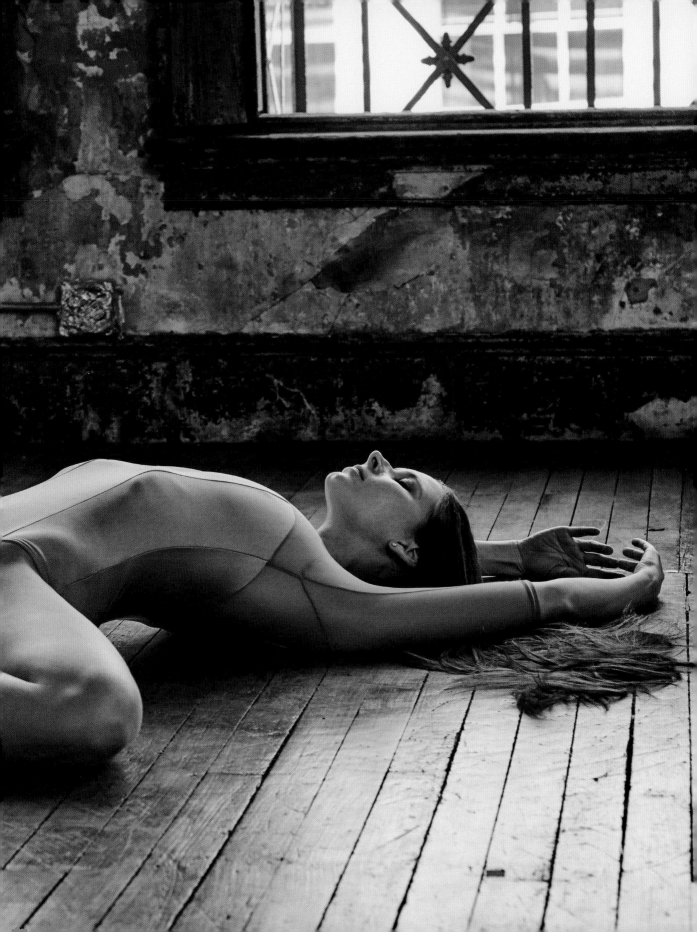

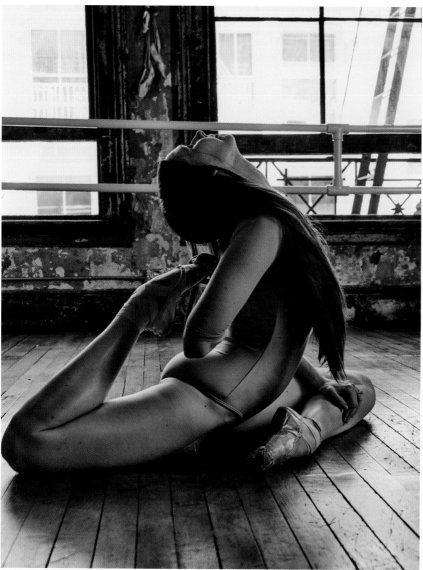

Hip stretch with *cambré derrière*.

Dance Principle
Frequent stretching of the quadriceps lengthens the lines of the legs while releasing tension through the hip flexors.

Pro Tip
This advanced stretch is most effective when the muscles are warm, so let it lead your cooldown stretch after a workout.

Fitness Tip
From a seated position with the front knee bent, bend the back knee and pull the toe up toward the shoulders, with the hip turned in parallel, opening through the hips and thighs. For a deeper stretch, lift up and arch with the upper body into a *cambré* back, pulling the toe toward the head. Take a deep breath and slowly release, and then change sides.

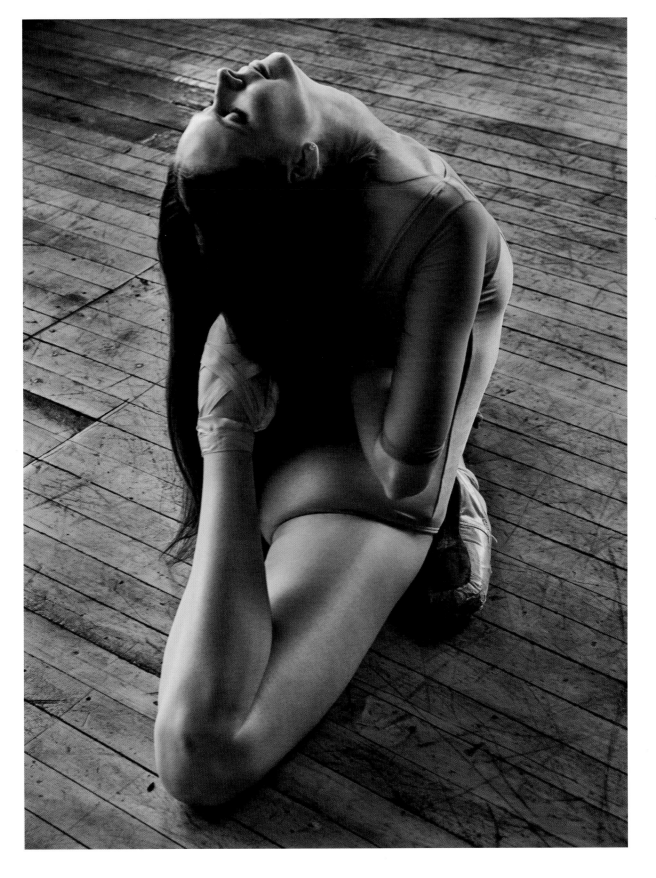

A Ballet Beautiful Body Flexibility

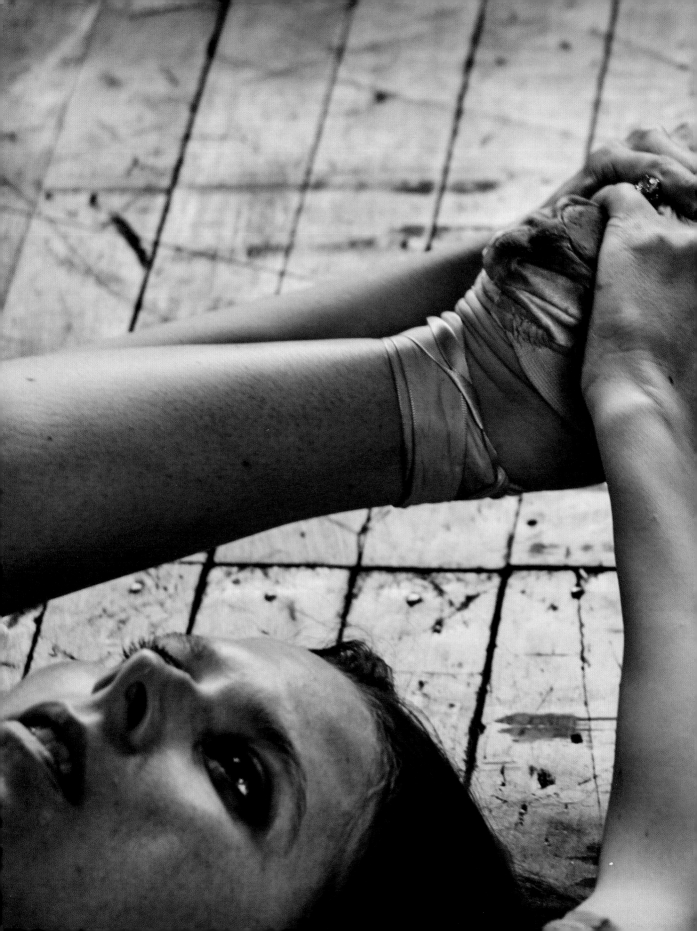

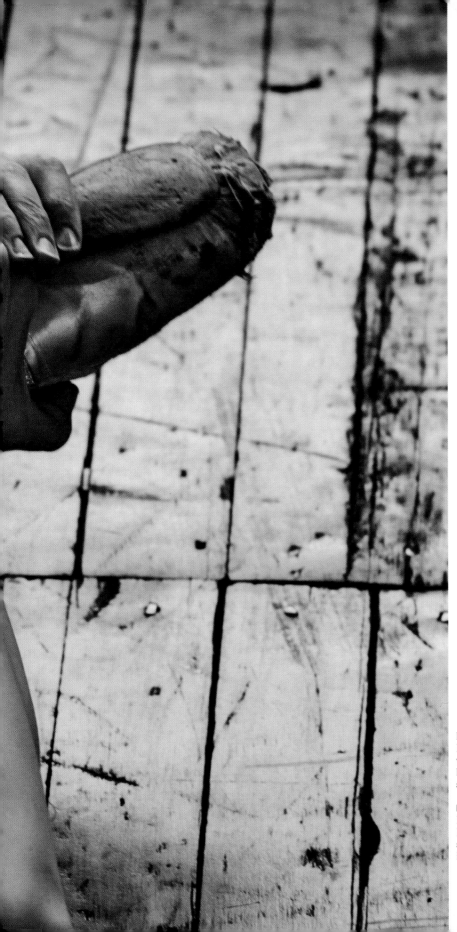

Dance Principle
Floor stretches are a wonderful way to work on increasing the extension of the legs for higher *battements*, *développés*, and *arabesques*.

Pro Tip
Flexibility can be increased over time. Find the limits of your range of motion and then work toward meeting and increasing your personal best each day.

143

PART 2

A
Beau

Ballet
tiful
Life

*M*y love for ballet has always extended beyond the stage, inspiring my wardrobe, workouts, and even my home. My closet is filled with peachy silks and muted blush tones reminiscent of my beloved pointe shoes. For me, the love story began when, as a girl, I met my first pair of toe shoes. I'll never forget the day my childhood ballet teacher Gay Porter told me that I was ready to begin training en pointe. Finally, the day had come for me to become a real ballerina! My mom and I drove across town so that I could get fitted for a pair of these magical shoes. That evening I hovered over her as she sewed on the ribbons at our kitchen table. I wore this pair until I outgrew them, and then hung them on the full-length cheval mirror in my childhood room, where they stayed until long after I was dancing in New York. That pair of tiny pink satin shoes flung open the doors to an enchanting new world.

Today I love blending my dancewear with everyday life. I practically live in my leotards, wearing them morning to evening, six or seven days a week. Whether I am training in the studio or not, leotards are the anchor of most of my outfits—I love how easy they are to layer over, the perfect canvas for a wide variety of everyday looks. Top them with a floaty maxi skirt or jean shorts in the summer or pencil skirts or wide-legged jeans in the fall. Just add seamed tights or legwarmers and a ballet skirt and you are ready for a workout!

Seeing the playful spin that others put on ballerina style makes dance fashion even more fun. Whether you are more sporty or classic in style, dance clothes offer something for everyone. A sports bra paired with a jersey skirt and tights or knit shorts reads "dancer" in a fresh and unexpected way, particularly when topped off with ballet slippers. And while a leotard and tights is an instant classic, leotards look equally as great when worn with leggings or with a floaty tulle skirt for a more romantic look, depending on your taste.

The same effortless ballet style applies to beauty routines. A simple bun is always chic, and paired with glowing skin makes for a timeless look. This is also an easy way to quickly take your workout look to the street. Whether in afternoon meetings or just running errands, an elegant updo and pink cheeks read: "I just left the ballet studio." The options for ballet-inspired hair are almost endless. I love the simplicity of a centered classic high or low bun, along with a more complicated French twist and fun low bun with a side part and braids. Fresh flowers or a ribbon add color and a feminine touch. Dress it up with eyeliner and red lipstick for more of an "onstage" look, or a simple smoky eye and nude gloss, depending on your mood.

The connection between diet and fitness is also an important one. Like workouts, a diet should also strengthen and power the body, from the inside out. Nevertheless, the pressure on a ballerina to be thin can be intense. Throughout the course of my career my weight has fluctuated and there have been times when I have felt at odds with my body rather than connected to it. In an effort to quickly lose weight, I experimented with crash dieting, no carbs, and other fads over the years. As my weight bounced up and down I eventually came to see that obsessing over my diet created more problems than it solved. Dieting made me miserable and insecure, and I was far from my healthiest. It was only after I began to relax about my diet and my figure that the pieces began to come together. I now know that my body works best when I treat it with care. This lesson has been an important part of the development of Ballet Beautiful, but getting there wasn't easy.

I have found that when I eat the right foods I don't obsess over portions, and, unlike some stringent diets, I never have to feel hungry. While I love a burger and fries as much as the next gal, I also love how great, healthy foods make me feel. I always feel better after a workout and the same is true after a healthy meal. Too much salt makes me bloated and wild with thirst. Heavy fried foods work only in moderation, so if I am having a serving of fried chicken, I pair it with a fresh spinach salad and berries for dessert. Overdoing sugary sweets makes my stomach ache, particularly before a workout. I like to think of fresh organic fruits and vegetables working as the building blocks for snacks and meals, and then I add in lean proteins, grains, and healthy fats like avocados and raw nuts. Rather than renouncing sweet treats entirely, I do indulge—in moderation. This helps to keep my eating on a healthy track and prevent overindulgence or any sort of "bingeing," because I feel satisfied and happy, rather than deprived. I cherish my tea in the afternoons (green tea with lemon or Earl Grey with organic milk, please) complemented by dark chocolate or gingersnaps, and, in the evenings before dinner, sharp cheese and red wine. If I'm prepping for an event or shoot and need to trim things back a bit, I might add in an extra salad during the day and cut the wine and cheese.

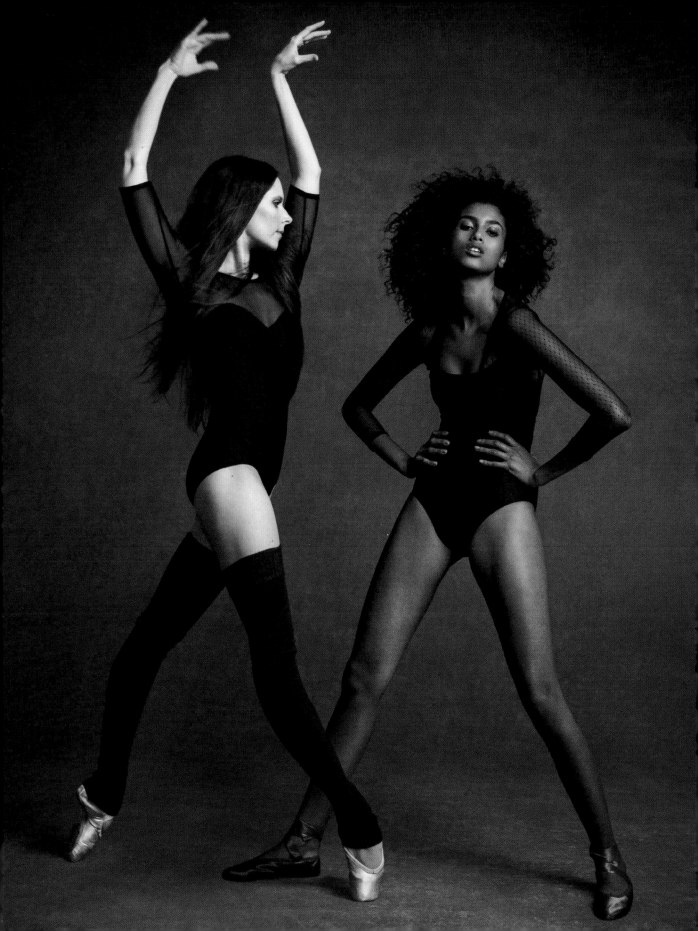

Style

*F*or ballet dancers, style is about melding personal expression with physical form. Embraced by celebrities and fashion icons like Audrey Hepburn, Brigitte Bardot, Natalie Portman, and Alexa Chung, ballet fashion has a glamorous history. Classic, formfitting clothes are cut to flatter and reveal, allowing for sleek silhouettes and optimal movement without giving too much away.

Dancewear offers a fun mix of function and whimsy. Ballet clothes are designed first with a dancer's performance in mind. From leotards to woolly knitwear, each piece has a purpose and a specific role in a dancer's wardrobe. Tights permit a wide range of motion and accent a dancer's lines, while a leotard-sans-tights look shows off the powerful muscles in a dancer's legs in the studio. A simple scoop-neck leotard highlights a ballerina's swanlike neck and elegant posture, both rooted in a powerful core. Long-sleeved leotards provide coverage and warmth for every *port de bras*. Simple chiffon wrap skirts offer a floaty, opaque layer over the hips and butt while displaying the legs. Tutus and tulle practice skirts add structure and formality while bringing the focus to the lower legs. Cozy legwarmers and knit shorts keep the muscles warm and hips loose during rehearsals and classes. A simple ballet wrap sweater heats the back muscles but is easy to put on or take off without disturbing a dancer's makeup or hair before a performance or during a workout.

I love the way that my dance clothes perform, both in the studio and out, from season to season. Classic pieces like ballet flats and soft wrap sweaters add elegance and ease to any look. When shopping for dresses, skirts, or the perfect pair of high-waisted jeans, I always think about how I can work in my leotards. Seamed ballet tights transition a look from summer to fall, as an easy layering piece for a workout as well as under almost any skirt or dress. Legwarmers over tights with boots or flats take that same look into the cold winter months. Ribboned satin and leather ballerina flats paired with jeans or A-line skirts make for the perfect off-duty-dancer look. I am often stopped on the street or subway when I am wearing my Ballet Beautiful flats. It's always fun when a mom points to my feet and tells her little one, "Look, a real ballerina!" Lumina, our older daughter, is completely mesmerized by ballet shoes, both hers and mine. Tutus are also one of her favorite fashion accessories, whether paired with tights and a sweater for a trip to the farmer's market or under a fancy dress, petticoat style. Lumina tells us, "I want to go to work with Mommy and climb the big stairs and wear ballet shoes." (Our SoHo studio is a fifth-floor walk-up and a serious heart-pumping climb!)

Designing and creating dance clothes has taken my love for dancewear to a whole other level, melding the creative process with my daily fashion and allowing me to bring my most dreamed-about ballet styles to life. Seeing these styles on others is the icing on the cake! Whether a top fashion editor in our NYC studio, a supermodel like Lily Aldridge, Doutzen Kroes, Miranda Kerr, or a Ballet Beautiful novice training with us online, witnessing our clients make ballet style their own inspires me to view ballet fashion through fresh eyes. Iconic beauty Raquel Zimmerman has a soft spot for a classically cut leotard and tulle, while model Imaan Hammam favors simple black camisoles with a pop of red in a satin shoe. Meanwhile, fashion It girls Harley Viera-Newton and Alexa Chung put their own unique stamp on ballerina street style, casually knotting the ribbons of their slippers and tossing them around their shoulders for a post-workout look that is always chic.

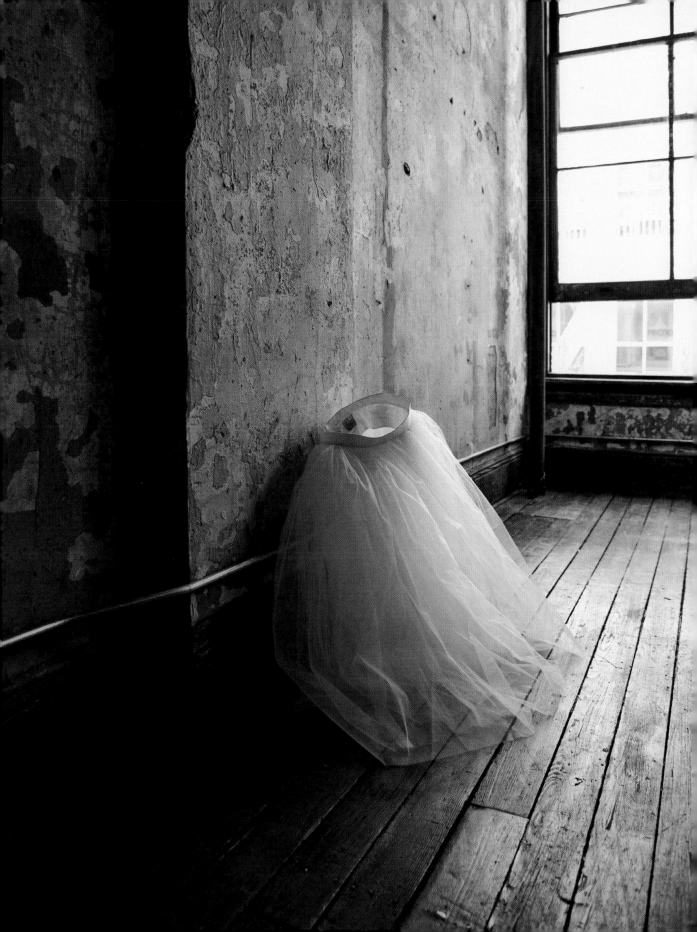

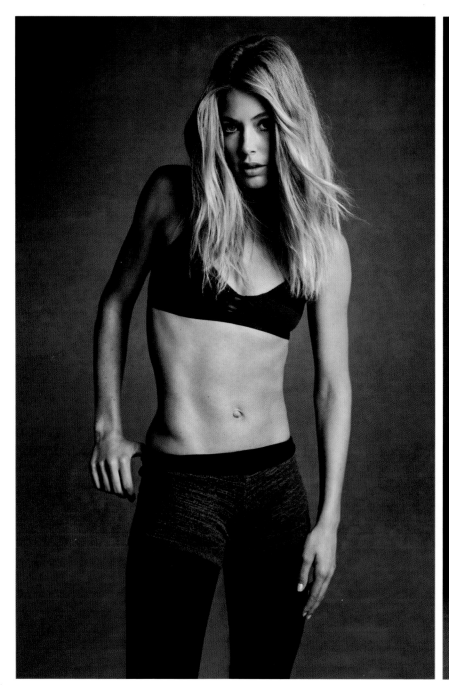

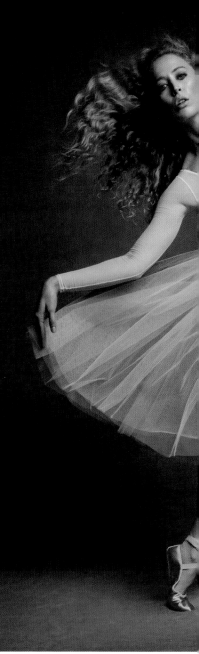

[PREVIOUS PAGE] A "romantic"-style practice tutu features a layered tulle skirt that falls past a dancer's knees. Practice tutus are tutus designed to be worn in rehearsals or in the studio over a leotard, without a bodice or as part of a larger costume.

Dance Principle

There are several different tutu styles. Longer, "romantic"-style tutus harken back to ballet's romantic era in the nineteenth century. World-renowned ballerinas like Marie Taglioni and Carlotta Grisi originated title roles in classical, full-length ballets like *La Sylphide* and *Giselle*. The shin-length tulle costume typical of these ballets was named in honor of this formative period for classical ballet.

Pro Tip

Pair a romantic practice tutu with a simple leotard or sports bra for a dreamy ballet-inspired workout look.

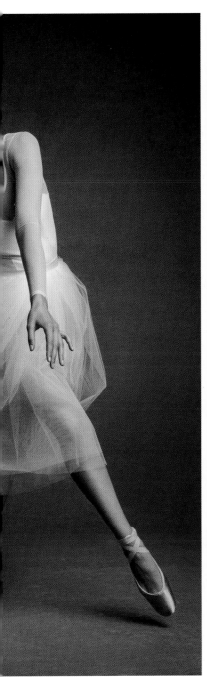

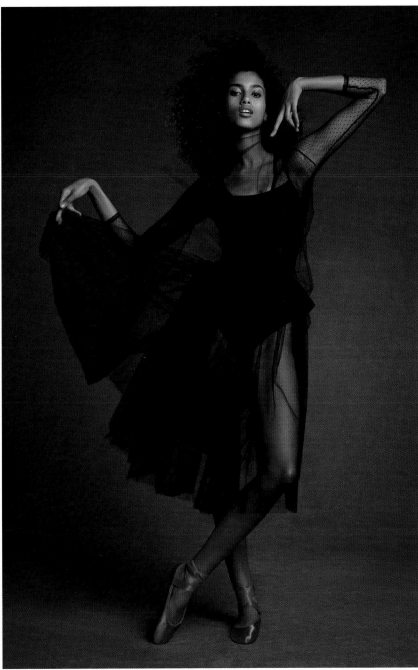

[THIS PAGE + OPPOSITE] Models Doutzen Kroes, Raquel Zimmermann, and Imaan Hammam make ballet style their own.

Dance Principle
Satin ballet slippers tied with ribbons provide the polished look of a pointe shoe with the comfort and accessibility of a soft-soled dance slipper.

Fitness Tip
Show off your ballerina abs with an athletic mix of a sports bra and leggings or seamed tights with shorts. Swap your leggings or tights for a romantic tutu's traditional ballet style and sheer coverage of the derrière and thighs.

A leotard with seamed tights or a simple chiffon skirt is a casual "in-the-studio" workout look.

Dance Principle

Leotards are a staple of a dancer's wardrobe, but they also offer a myriad of styling possibilities. Seamed tights are typically worn over the entire foot and inside of pointe or soft shoes during performances, but in class and rehearsals anything goes. Cutting the toes and feet of tights provides a range of styling options for a ballerina's look.

Pro Tip

Wear your leotard underneath a pair of black or pink seamed ballet tights for an authentic pro look, or with bare legs and a classic wrap skirt or hot pants for a more athletic style. Pulling the tights down over the heel of the shoe (pictured, below) lengthens the line of the leg. A second cut along the heel creates a stirrup that allows for the same visual effect with better traction. Bare legs draw the eye to a dancer's muscles, highlighting power and muscle tone.

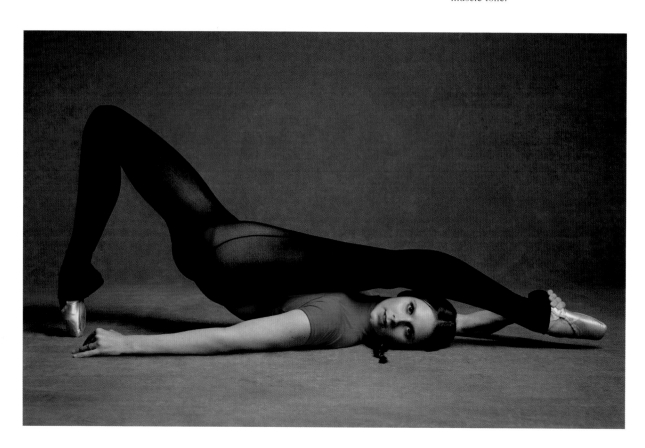

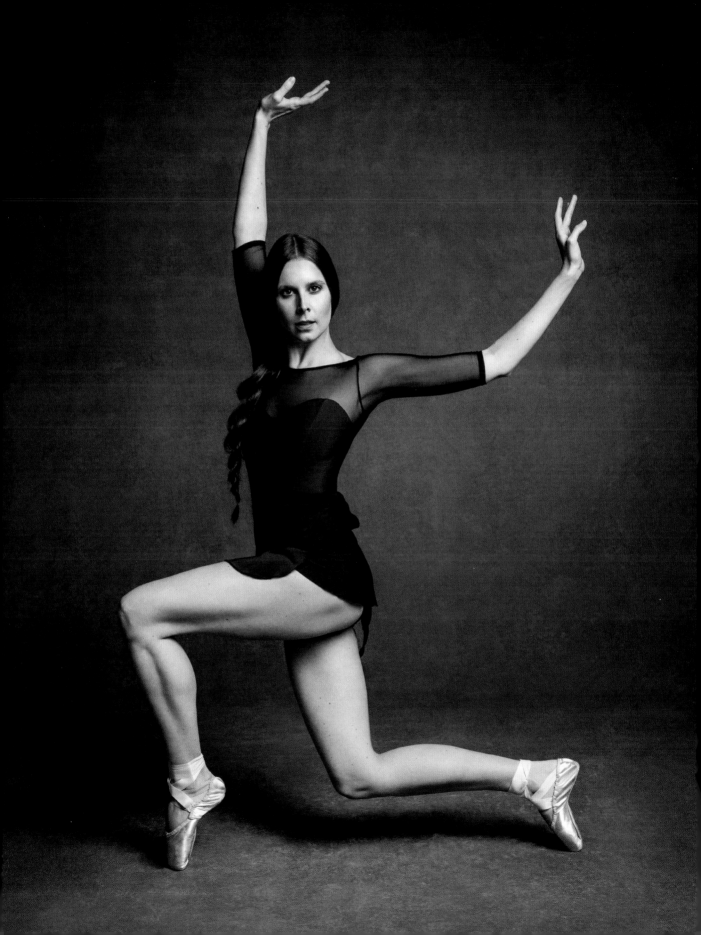

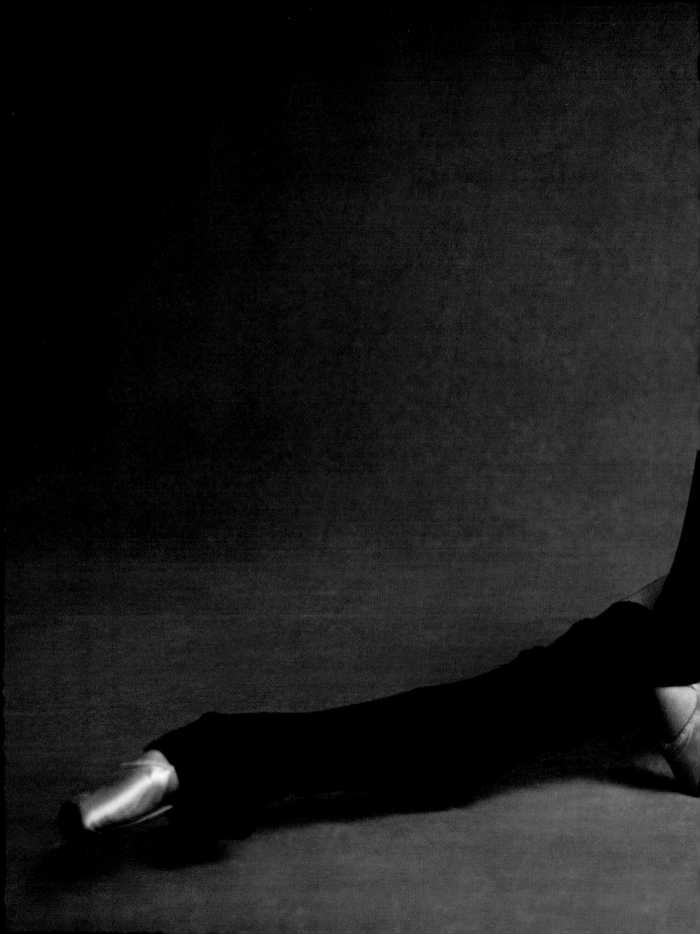

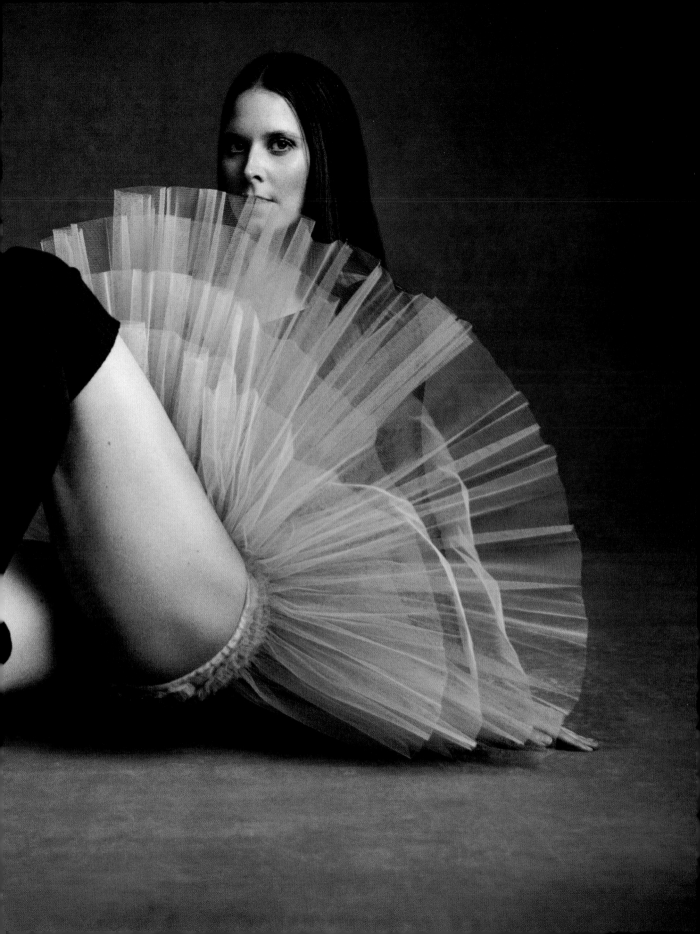

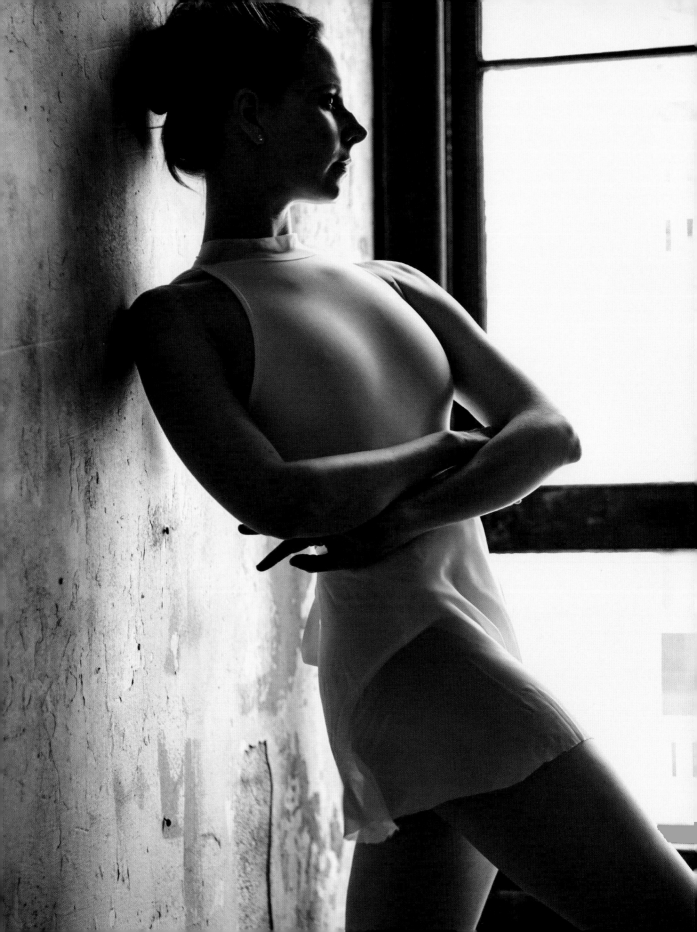

[PREVIOUS PAGES] A classic or "pancake"-style tutu includes a ruffled, tulle brief with graduated layers of tulle that stand straight out from the hips.

Dance Principle

Pancake-style tutus are typical of full-length, classical ballets like Swan Lake and the Nutcracker along with George Balanchine's neoclassical Symphony in C.

Fitness Tip

Pair a classic practice tutu with a scoop-neck leotard and bare legs for sporty yet feminine ballerina style. Layer thigh-high legwarmers over leggings or tights to keep the muscles warm.

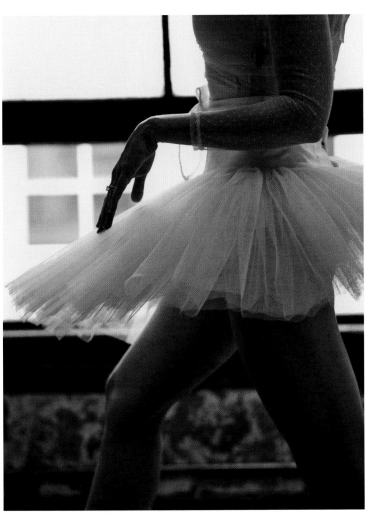

[OPPOSITE + THIS PAGE] Feminine details like a chiffon wrap skirt and pancake tutu with a mesh wrap top draw attention to the lines of a dancer's legs while providing coverage of the derrière, hips, and upper thighs.

Pro Tip

Buy a long chiffon skirt and trim with sharp scissors to personalize the length.

Fitness Tip

A halter-neck leotard is ideal for cardio workouts, showing off back muscles and beautiful posture while keeping the arms and shoulders cool. A mesh wrap top provides breathability in a lightweight, stretchy layer.

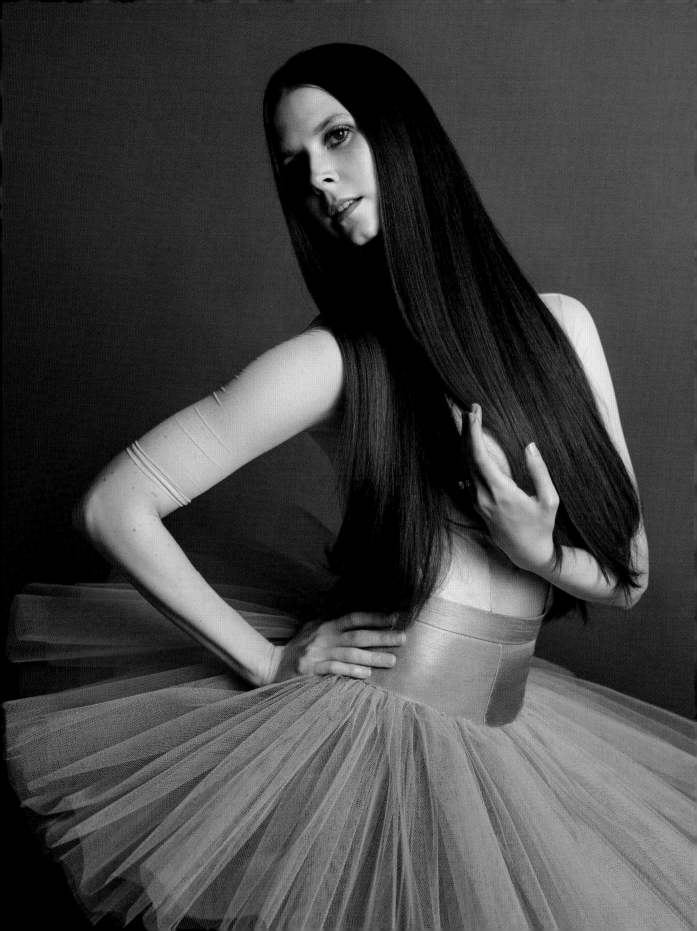

2.2

Beauty

*B*eauty is an inherent part of every ballerina's daily routine. Carefully sculpted chignons, winged eyeliner, and glowing skin are classic beauty looks that translate seamlessly from the studio to the stage and beyond.

For a dancer, hair and makeup complete every look without detracting from the body's line or movement. Hair is always pulled back so it's out of the face for daily class and rehearsals, often pinned into a simple bun. For performances, hair styles are often dictated by the ballets themselves. For example, classic, full-length ballets like *Swan Lake* and *Gisele* require dancers to wear their hair in a low bun whereas dancers in Balanchine's neoclassical "leotard ballets" and his *Symphony in C* wear a sleek high bun. Dancers' hair is loose for Balanchine's *Chaconne* and *Tschaikovsky Suite No. 3*, while the ballerinas in *Apollo* and *Mozartiana* require a high bun with pinned-on curls. Meanwhile, each ballerina in *Symphony in Three Movements* pulls her hair back in a high, swingy ponytail. The variations within each bun can be endless. Braids, twists, and loops are all personal favorites. Onstage looks require extra hair pins and products to secure every loose flyaway and headpiece—hairspray and gels are required. French hair pins of different sizes help to hold a bun in place without flattening its shape and are a staple of my beauty kit. Forget triple pirouettes—to me, there are few things more satisfying than achieving a perfectly smooth high ponytail at the first attempt.

Most dancers do their own hair and makeup, making the approach very DIY. I'll never forget my confusion at my first performance with New York City Ballet over how to do my hair and makeup for the stage. In the days leading up to that performance I made a quick trip to the drugstore to purchase stage makeup with a friend who had performed in the School of American Ballet's workshop the summer before. But once I was sitting in the dressing room backstage before that performance, I found I had no idea how to apply the false lashes, liquid liner, or the heavy pancake foundation used for stage! When my requests for help from some of the older girls in the dressing room were turned down, I checked in with the younger girls for tips and went at it on my own. I worked off instinct and memories of beloved old dance photographs and just tried to follow along. That night my beauty look was not my most professional, but I quickly learned how to line my eyes, apply contouring, blush, red lips, and powder to make the most of my features for an audience of thousands.

When it comes to my beauty routine for workouts, I like to mix it up. After years of pulling my hair into super-tight buns onstage, I now favor a more relaxed look in the studio. I often pin my hair up without using a hair band, or I pull it into a long, loose braid. Fresh flowers or even a simple pointe-shoe ribbon or piece of chiffon adds a dash of fancy. With makeup, I like a day-to-day look that is more low-key: clean skin with just a touch of concealer, highlighter, and blush for a natural, dewy glow. I tend to wear mascara only when shooting, in meetings, or out at night. For a more dramatic onstage look I like heavy liquid eyeliner and mascara on the top and bottom.

[OPPOSITE] Clean skin and softly lined eyes make for a toned-down version of classical ballet stage makeup in everyday life.

[FOLLOWING PAGES] Tortoiseshell accessories, a wide tooth comb, and French hair pins are staples of a chic ballerina up-do.

Dance Principle
French hair pins (bottom right) are designed to hold the hair in place in an intricate bun or twist. The pins are long and thin, reaching deep within the bun to secure the hair without disturbing the style.

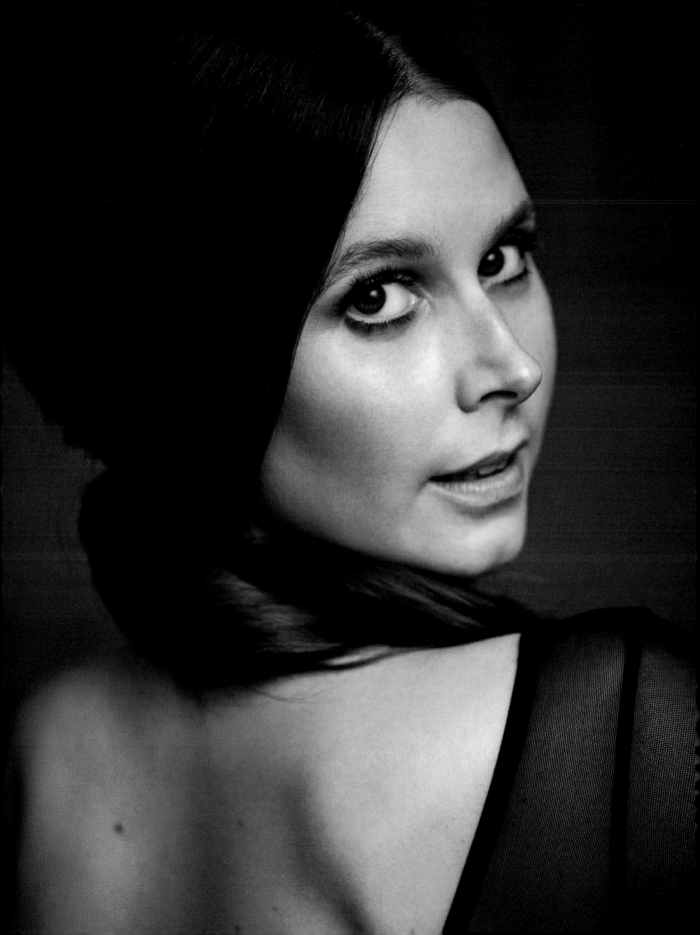

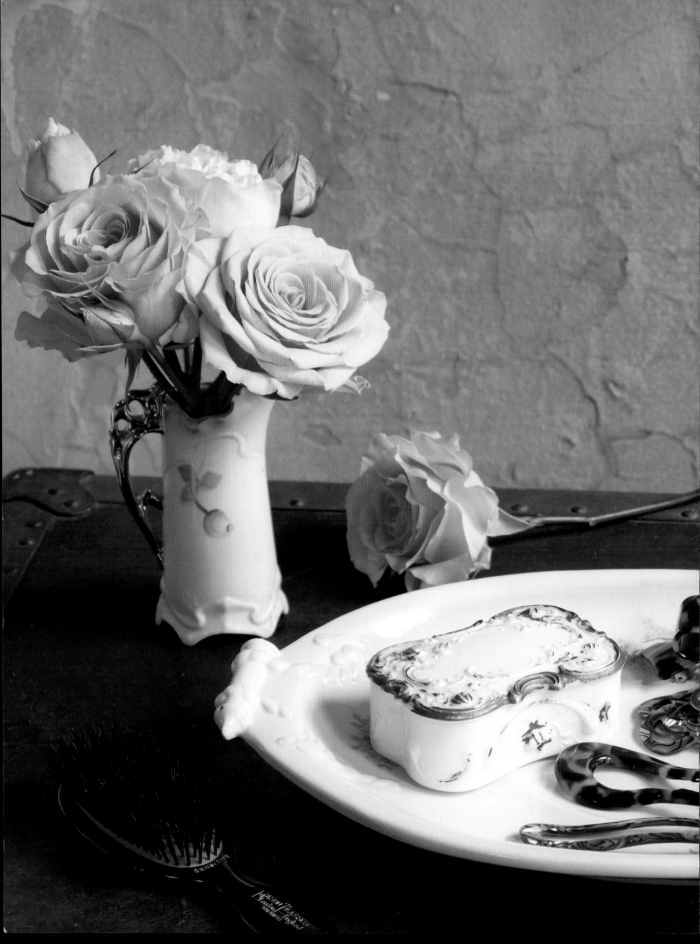

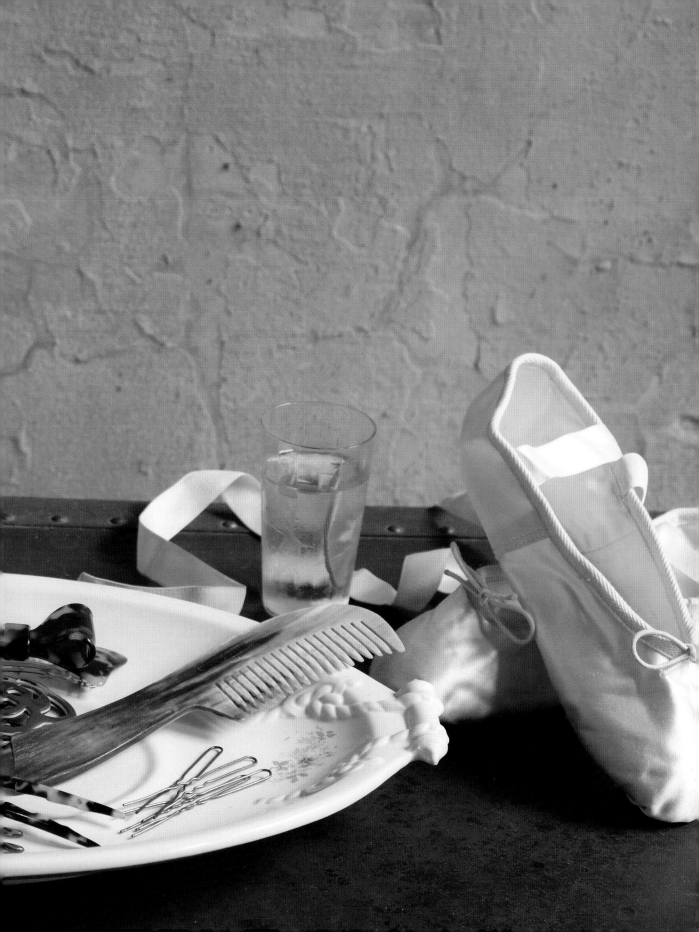

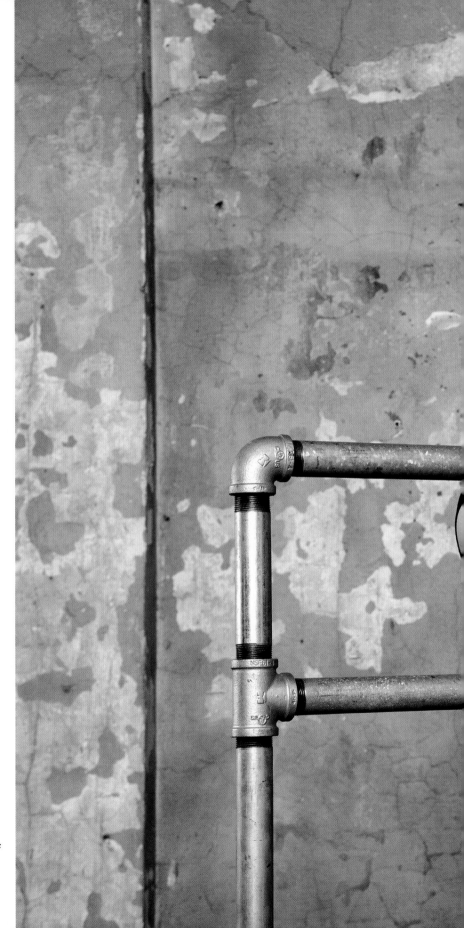

A bold, smoky eye stands out in the studio or on stage. Pair with glowing skin and a nude lip gloss for a beauty look that is all about the eyes.

Dance Principle
Fresh skin and big eyes epitomize classic ballerina style, reminiscent of Balanchine ballerinas like Suzanne Farrell and Patricia McBride.

Pro Tip
Top your eyeshadow with a touch of clear lip gloss for extra shine. Keep the lips and cheek neutral to make the eyes pop.

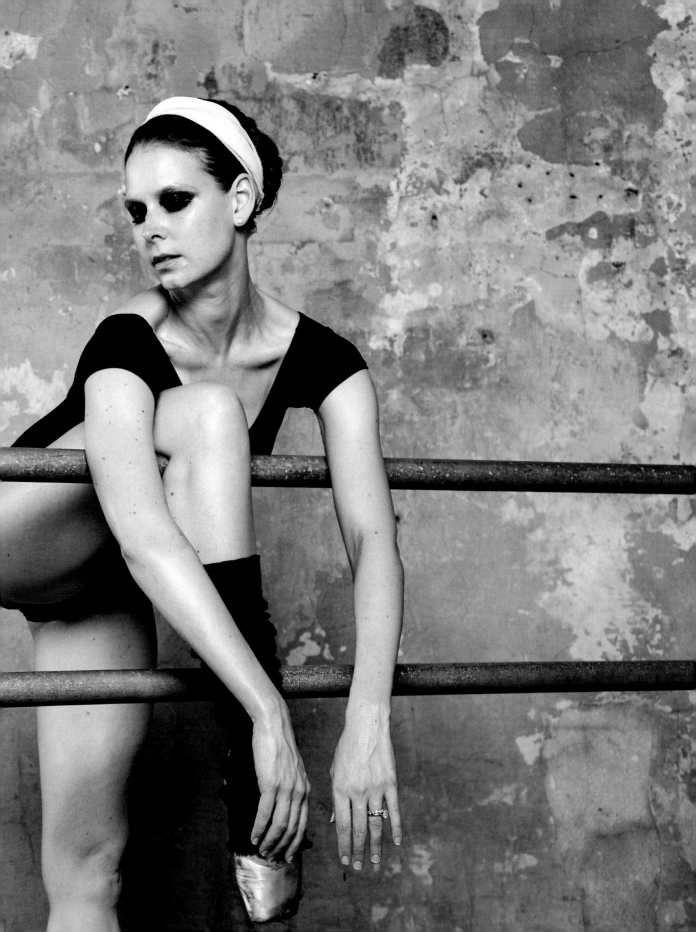

An intricate braided bun with a chiffon wrap and a messy loose bun are elegant variations on classic ballerina style.

Pro Tip

When onstage, sleek hair is a requirement. Tight hairbands and ponytail holders, gel, water, hair spray, and hairpins secure the hairstyle and headpieces, no matter the movement. For a workout or rehearsal with a more relaxed look, simply twist the hair into a bun, pin, and go!

[THIS PAGE]

Pro Tip

Create your own headband by cutting a small piece of chiffon (this piece was taken from the bottom of a dance skirt, see page 158) and wrapping it around your bun. Secure the look with a few bobby pins.

Fitness Tip

A cloth headband keeps the hair out of the face, allowing you to focus on your workout, not your hair.

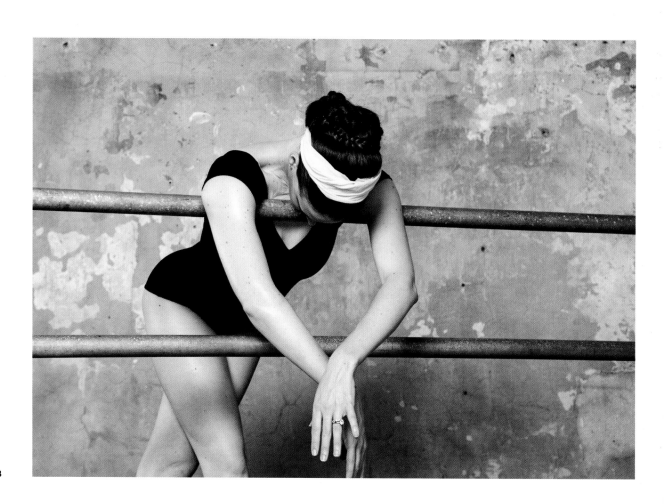

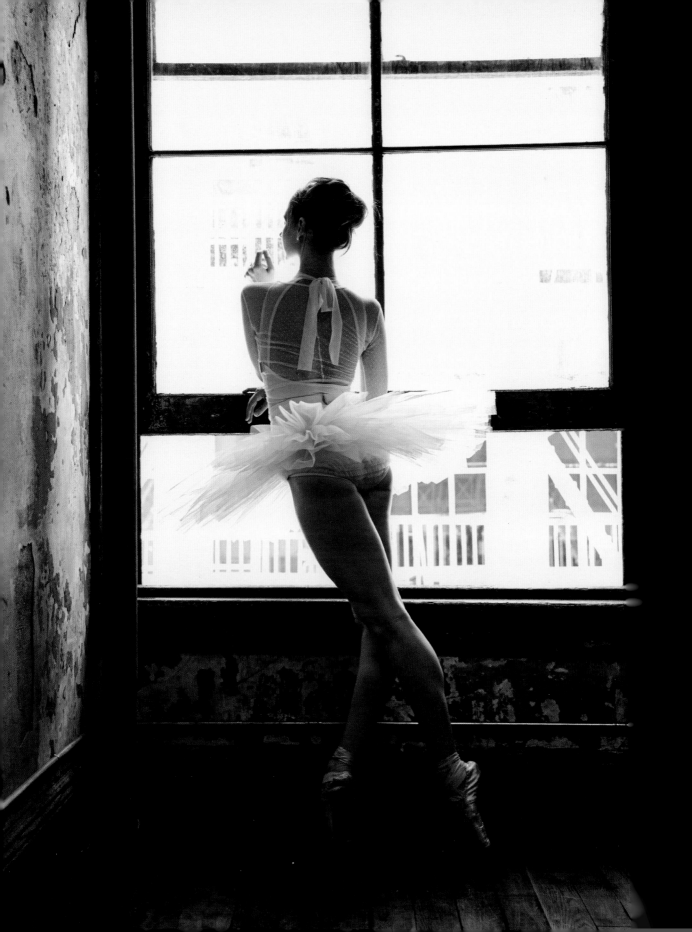

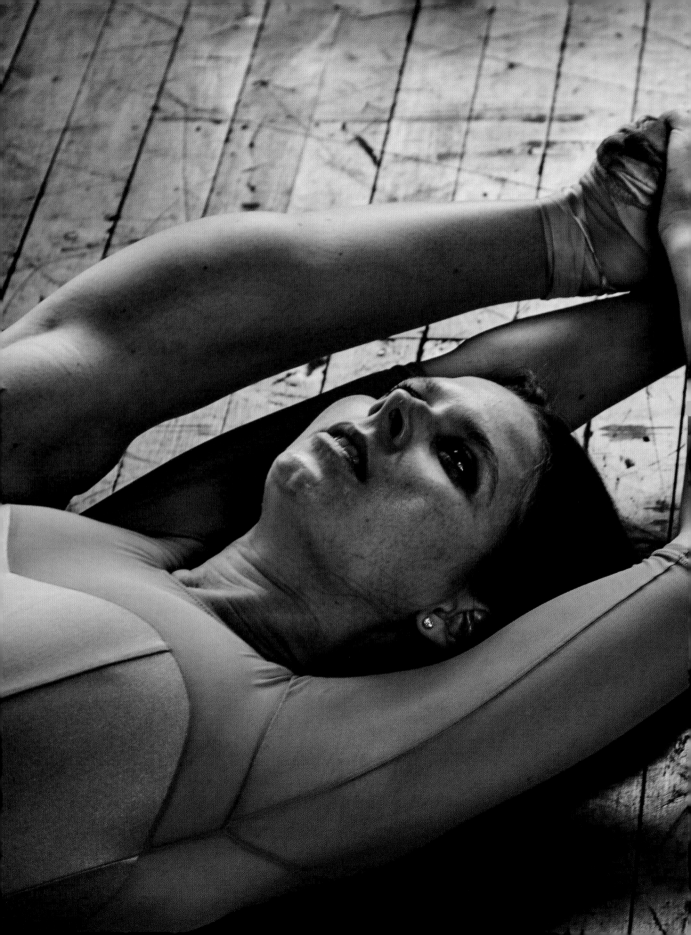

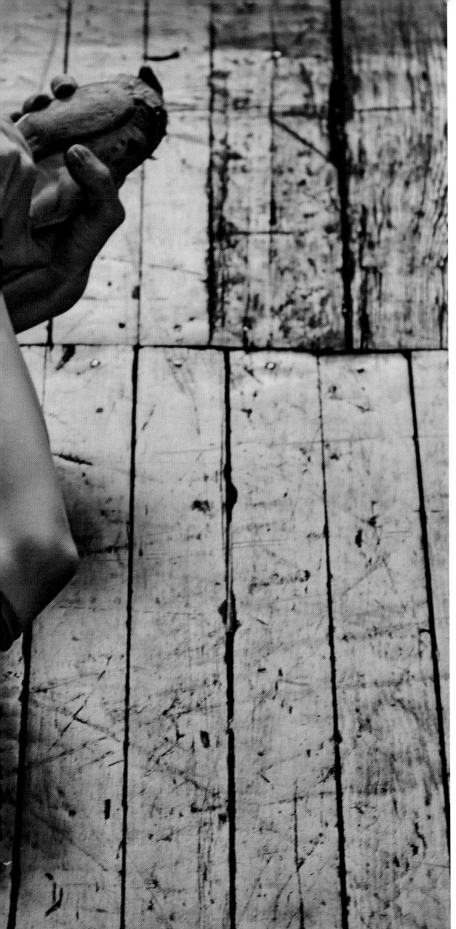

Clean, glowing skin and loose hair make for a relaxed, "I just finished my workout" look.

Dance Principle
This "offstage" look makes the occasional appearance onstage. Balanchine ballets like *Chaconne* and the "Elegy" section of Brahms's *Schoenberg Quartet* include "hair down" sections with loose, flowing hair.

Pro Tip
When it comes to glowing skin, less makeup is more. Skip the foundation and powder to let your natural glow shine through. A great concealer mixed with a low-shine highlighter on the brows and cheekbones conceals dark circles while a workout provides the perfect shade of natural blush.

171

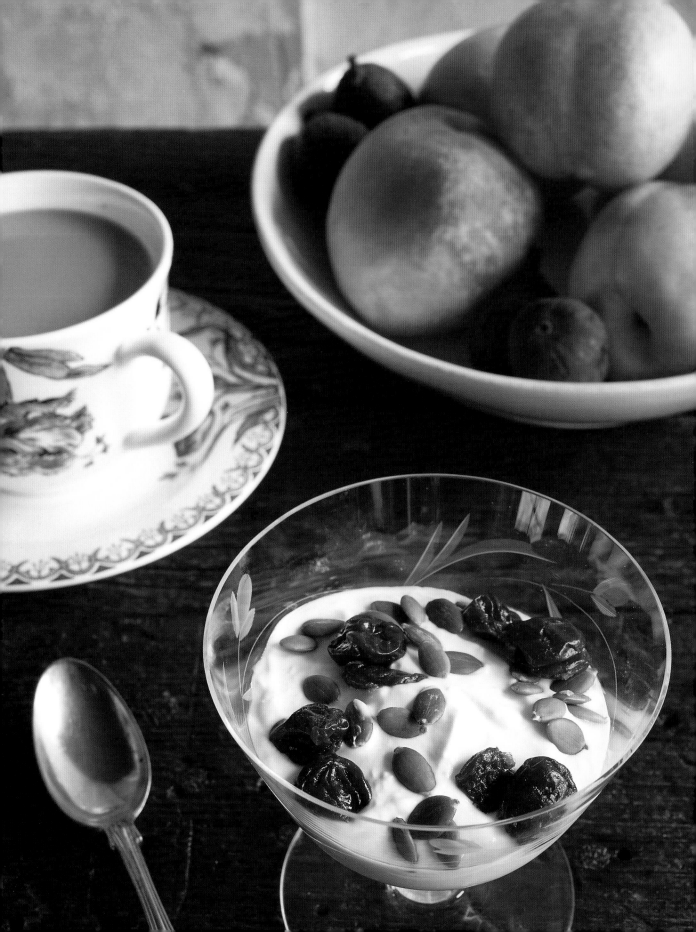

2 . 3

Kitchen

A Ballet Beautiful kitchen is filled with foods that nourish the body and support a beautiful, healthy glow. Fresh local produce, lean proteins like grilled salmon and chicken and organic yogurts, and complex carbs are our staples. The Ballet Beautiful approach to healthy eating is to focus on quality ingredients without a lot of fuss. Delicious, satisfying meals and snacks provide energy and colorful inspiration for my workouts and everyday life.

I enjoy cooking but, like most of us, I am often running short on time. I'm not a strict recipe person, but being able to prepare meals at home helps me keep on top of the ingredients my family and I are consuming. Keeping my fridge and pantry stocked with healthy choices that can serve as building blocks for meals helps me to stay committed to simple, healthy, meals at home. When I go shopping, I start with produce. While I may have a certain meal in mind, I try to stay flexible, working with whatever seems the freshest. For example, rather than obsessing over finding the perfect head of broccoli rabe or Swiss chard, I pick whichever leafy green looks most enticing that day. This gives me more flexibility with my shopping list and ensures more variety in my diet, too; it is so easy to fall into a repetitive rut with grocery shopping and eating! Sometimes just trying a new variation on an old recipe does the trick for spicing up a favorite meal.

When buying produce, I try to always include fresh lettuce for salads in the warmer months and greens for soups in the winter and fall. In the summer, when local lettuce is in season, I buy double my usual amount and have two salads a day, with eggs on the weekend and again at dinner or lunch. I look for root vegetables like sweet potatoes as complex carbs year-round. I love red new potatoes served with olive oil and parsley in summer months. I might shred raw carrots and slice radishes into summer salads and roast carrots with Brussels sprouts, garlic, and walnuts in fall and winter. Fruit should be bought in season, too. Organic, local apples and pears are staples in the winter and fall, along with citrus. I love to start my morning with half a grapefruit in the cooler months for an extra boost of vitamin C. Berries of all descriptions and stone fruits like nectarines, apricots, and peaches along with melons are must-haves in the summer!

I find that when I am working out daily, my muscles require a fair amount of protein. Grilled, roasted, or baked chicken is a favorite along with fish like wild salmon. I eat red meat in moderation along with plenty of legumes like chickpeas, lentils, and beans for plant-based protein as well as variety. I do indulge in the occasional burger (I love to swap in spinach or salad in place of fries!) and I pair my steak with steamed or sautéed spinach and baked sweet potatoes to balance things out. Whole-grain pastas, brown rice, and quinoa all make healthy sides. For breakfast, slow-cooked oatmeal has been a staple of mine for years; I top it with raw walnuts or almonds and fresh fruit. Snacks might include fresh fruit with a boiled egg or Greek yogurt for extra protein. Organic coffee is a daily pleasure that I forgo only when pregnant. And, of course, we can't forget about my chocolate stash. I love dark chocolate, and keep multiple bars in my fridge at all times.

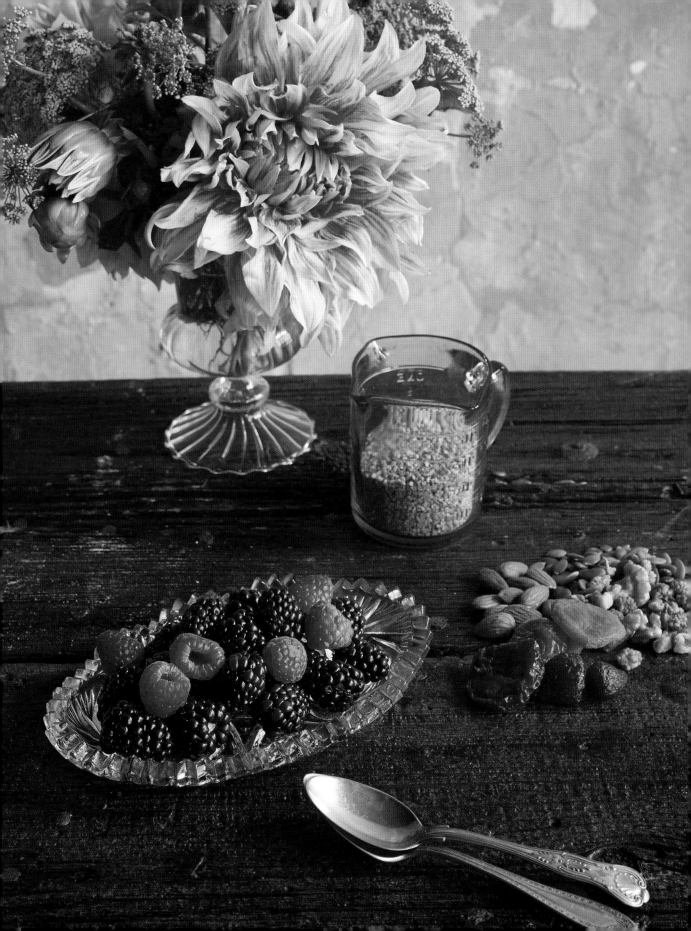

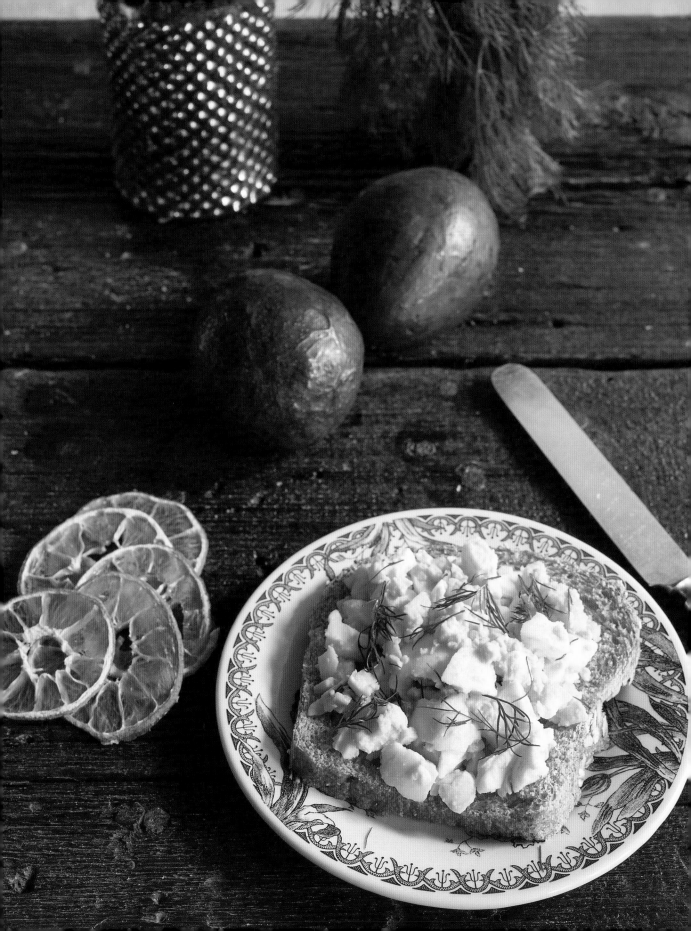

[PREVIOUS PAGES]
Whole grains, like steel-cut oatmeal
mixed with fresh berries and assorted
seeds and nuts, are great for a balanced
breakfast built around complex carbs
and healthy fats. Make an extra-large
pot of oatmeal and store in the fridge to
save time in the mornings or for healthy
evening snack.

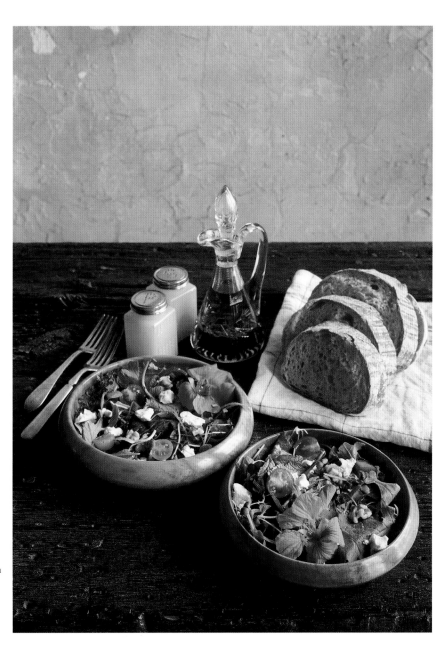

[OPPOSITE] Mashed boiled eggs with
olive oil and fresh dill are an excellent
option for a quick and easy mini-meal.
Serve on a slice of whole grain toast
for a healthy breakfast or filling
pre-workout snack packed with protein
and fiber.

[THIS PAGE] Goat cheese and walnuts
add fat, protein, and flavor to a simple
green salad.

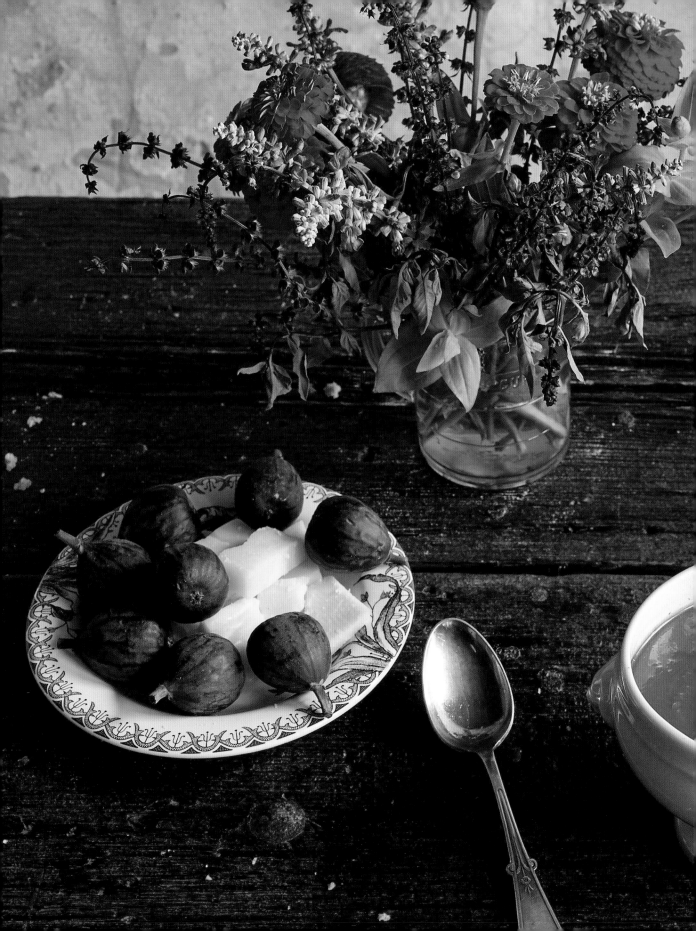

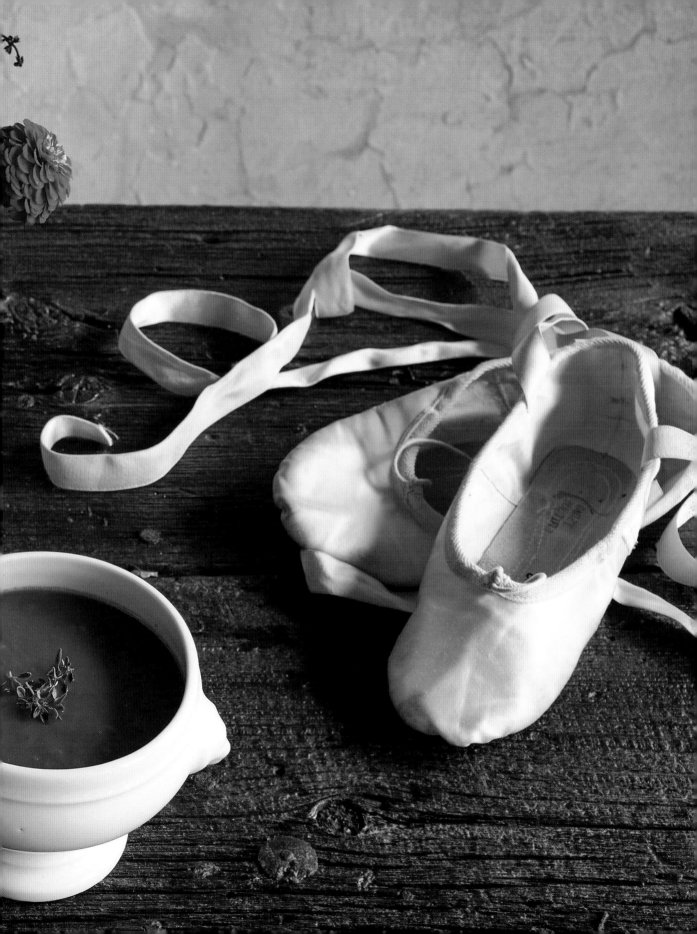

[PREVIOUS PAGES] Vegetarian soups, like this light cream-based tomato soup, and fruit and cheese combine for a light yet satisfying post-workout meal.

[THIS PAGE] Staying hydrated is a huge part of our health, keeping our digestion on track, helping to fight fatigue and providing a healthy glow from the inside out. Keep a glass or bottle of water with you and sip frequently during and after every workout. Add fresh fruit like berries or lemon slices to flavor naturally. Cucumbers and mint (pictured) turn a glass of regular water into a hydrating spa experience.

[OPPOSITE] Feeding your body high-quality protein, such as wild-caught salmon with fresh organic greens, keeps the metabolism humming.

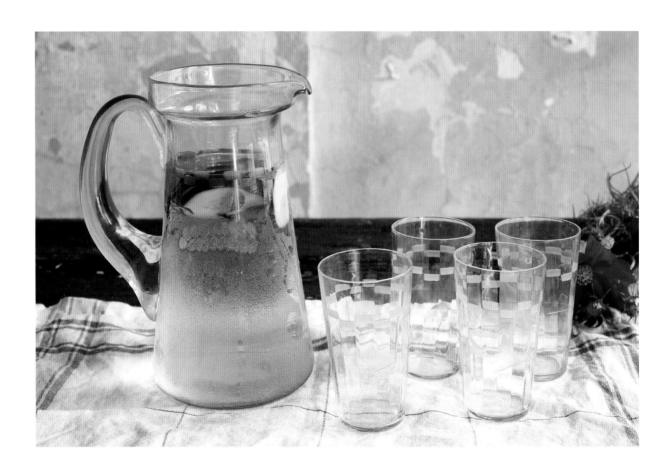

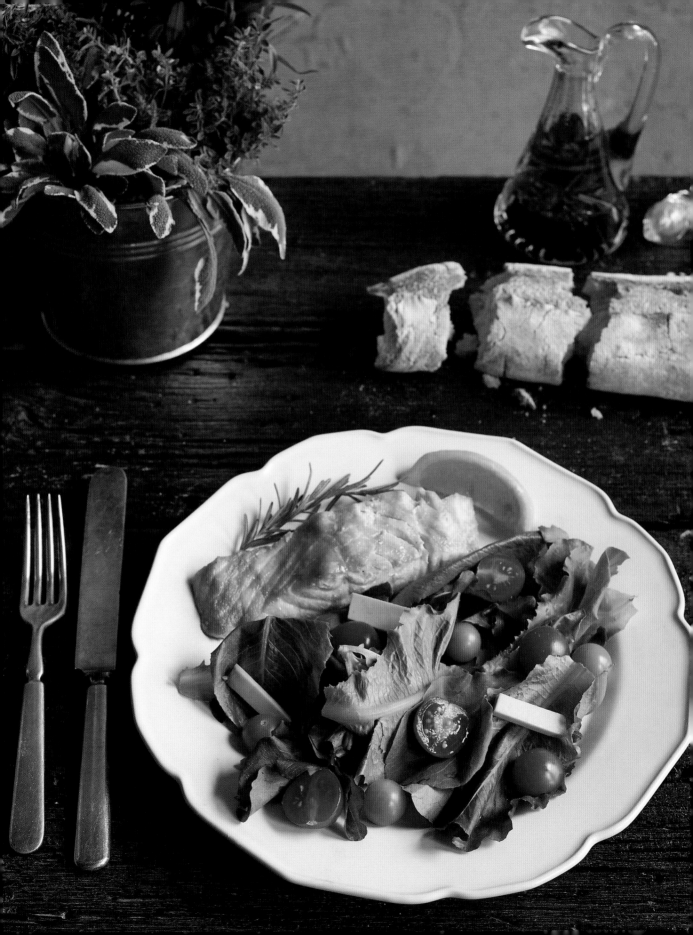

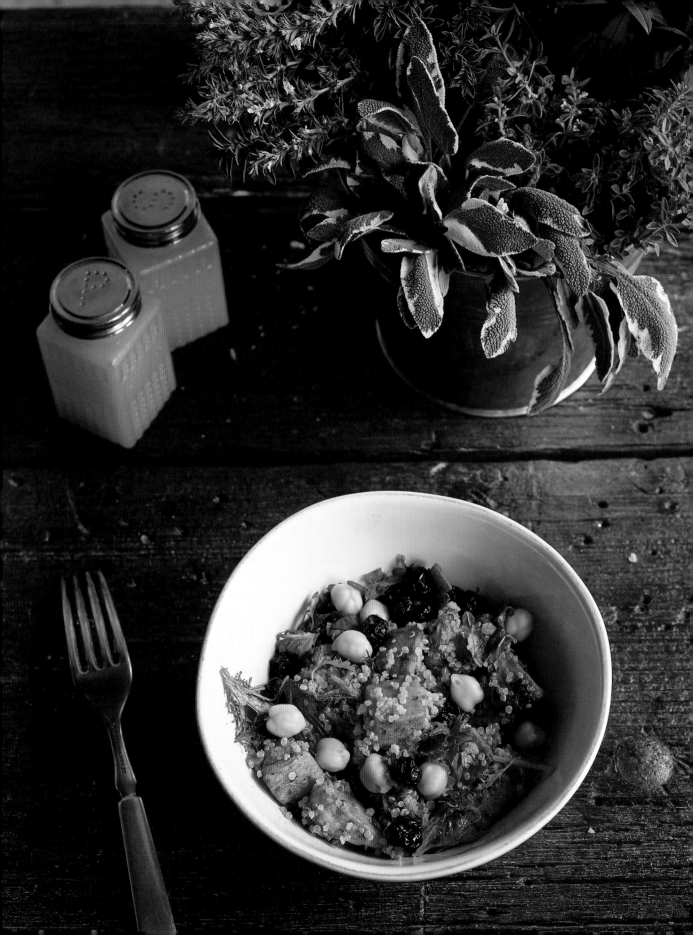

[OPPOSITE] Sweet potatoes and quinoa provide enduring energy and a slow burn. Add fresh greens, chick peas, and unsweetened, dried cherries for a satisfying plant-based salad and meal.

[THIS PAGE] Raw nuts, dark chocolate and dried and fresh fruit make for an energizing, healthy afternoon snack. After a workout a light snack can help the body build lean muscle and satisfy cravings. Raw, unsalted nuts provide healthy fats and protein while the fiber from an apple or a few pieces of dried fruit help to curb the appetite while delivering anti oxidants. A piece or two of dark chocolate with a small cup of tea or coffee satisfies sweet cravings. Keep apples and a small bag of raw nuts on you to stay satisfied and prevent yourself from getting too hungry after a workout or on the go.

[FOLLOWING PAGES] Hot tea and gingersnaps are a just-sweet-enough midday treat. Indulging in favorite treats in moderation keeps me satisfied and on track with healthy eating.

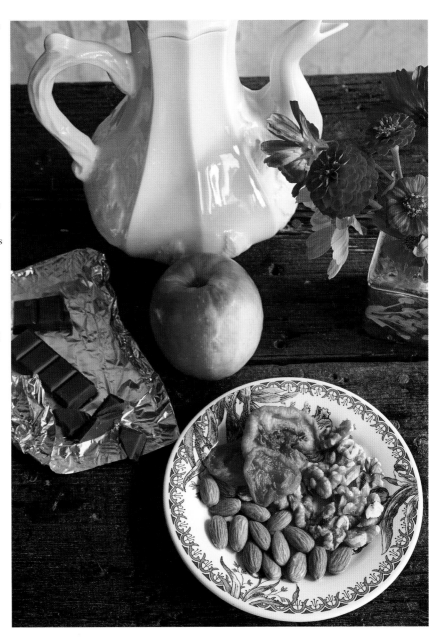

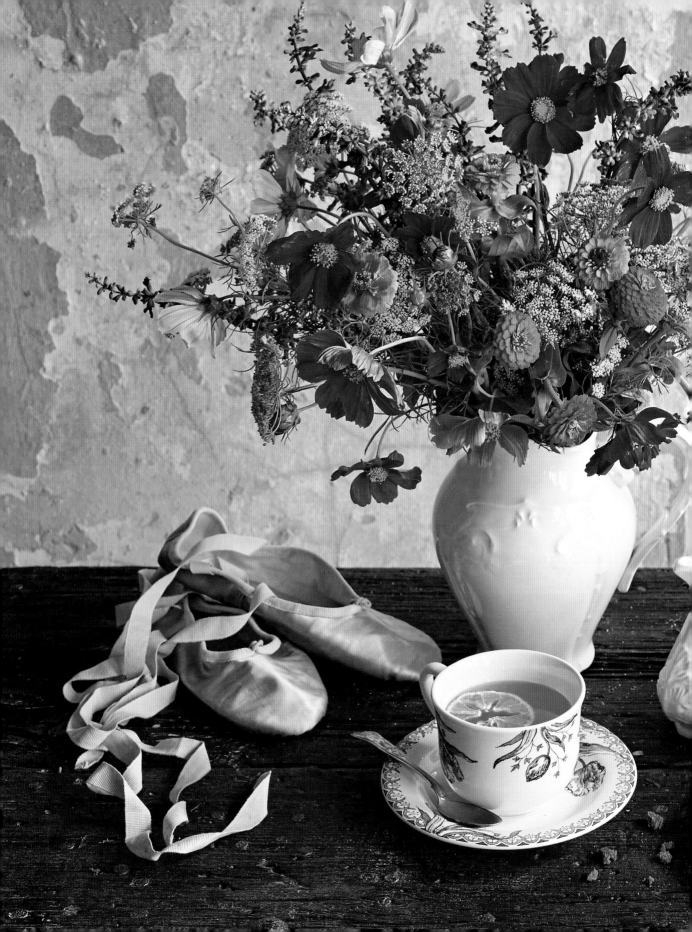

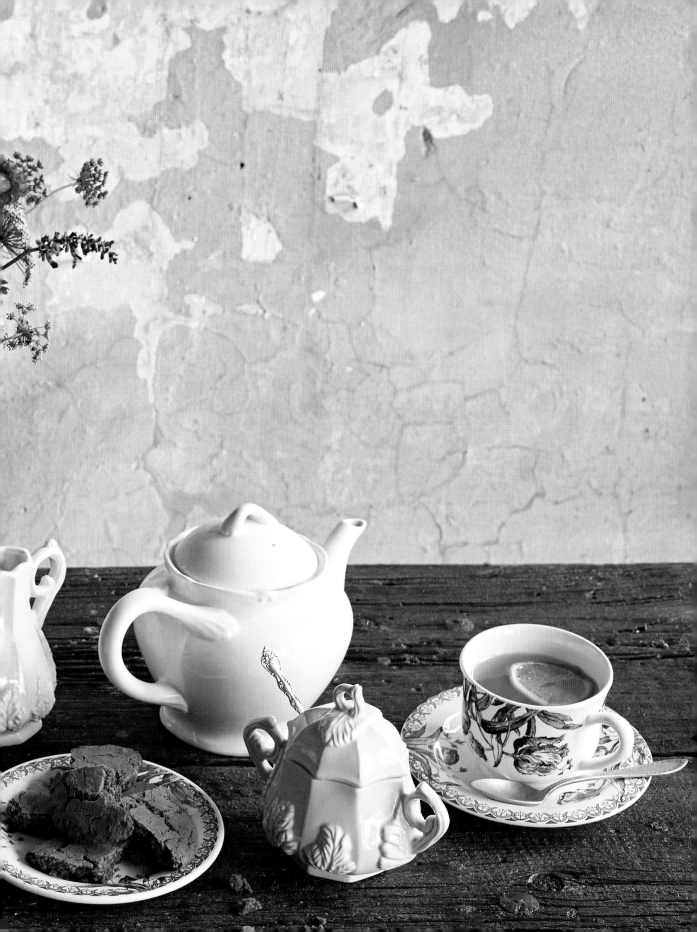

Glossary

Arabesque one of the classical positions in ballet, where the working leg is fully straight extending long behind the dancer either on the floor (*à terre*) or in the air (*en l'air*). The supporting (standing) leg can be straight or in a *demi-plié*. An *arabesque* can be performed in several variations: first, second, third, or fourth *arabesque*. The variations are based on the position of the arms, which create the longest line from the fingers to the toes.

First Arabesque when the dancer is standing in the *arabesque* position with the supporting leg straight or in *plié* and the working leg stretched long behind them, either on the floor or lifted off the ground. Extend the same arm as the leg behind to the side or at a slight diagonal back, and extend the same arm as the supporting leg out in front at shoulder height or slightly higher.

Second Arabesque beginning in the *arabesque* position with the legs. Extend the same arm as the leg behind in front, either at shoulder height or slightly higher, and the arm of the standing leg out to the side or at a slight diagonal back in second position.

Third Arabesque begin in the *arabesque* position with both arms extended to the front with both elbows straight. The arm on the same side as the standing leg should be lifted so that the hand is in line with the top of the head. The arm on the side of the leg in *arabesque* should be in line with the shoulder or slightly lower. The arms should be about a foot apart.

Fourth Arabesque with the dancer in an *arabesque* position, the arm of the supporting leg is extended forward with the fingertips slightly higher than the shoulder. The arm of the leg in *arabesque* is extended diagonally back behind the shoulder to match the line of the leg in *arabesque*.

Assemblé meaning "joined together" or "assembled." The basic form of an *assemblé* is when two legs join together in the air. One foot brushes off the ground as the dancer pushes off to ground to jump and have the supporting leg meet the brushed leg in the air in fifth position.

Attitude a classical ballet position where the working leg is lifted in the air to the front (*devant*), side (*à la seconde*), or to the back (*derrière*). The leg in the air is bent at a ninety-degree angle and is usually turned out so that the knee is higher than the foot. The supporting leg is straight, on pointe or *demi-pointe*.

Cambré meaning "arched." A *cambré* is a bend from the waist with the upper body arching forward, backward, or sideways with the arms following and completing the movement.

Cou-de-Pied meaning "on the 'neck' of the foot." *Cou-de-pied* is a position of the feet, where the working foot is pointed and placed on the standing leg between the base of the calf and the top of the ankle.

Cou-de-pied can be performed in two different variations, basic or wrapped. In basic cou-de-pied devant (to the front), the small toes of the pointed foot are placed in front of the supporting leg just above the top of the ankle. Basic cou-de-pied derrière (to the back) is performed with the heel of the pointed foot placed between the calf muscle and top of the ankle, this time behind the supporting leg. In a wrapped cou-de-pied, the heel of the pointed foot is placed in the front of the supporting leg with the foot wrapping around the ankle and the toes are behind reaching toward the floor.

Dégagé meaning "to disengage." *Dégagé* is a movement where the working leg "disengages" from the supporting leg. The working leg brushes off the floor extending in a fully stretched leg with a pointed foot to the front, side, or back of the supporting leg.

Grand Battement meaning "large beat." A ballet movement that is done by brushing the working leg off the floor, typically past ninety degrees, into the air before bringing it back to the starting position with control. *Grands battements* can be performed to the front (*devant*), side (*à la seconde*), or back (*derrière*).

Jeté meaning "throwing" or "thrown." A *jeté* is a type of jump from one foot to the other where the dancer brushes the working leg off the floor, jumping from the supporting leg and landing on the working leg. A *jeté* can be performed in many different variations.

Passé meaning "passed." A *passé* is performed when the working leg bends and passes along the supporting leg, forming a triangle shape with the toes either in front, to the side, or behind the knee of the supporting leg. The term *passé* is often used interchangeably with *retiré*.

Petit Battement meaning "small beat." A petit battement is a rapid beating movement of the working leg and foot around the ankle of the supporting leg. The working knee is bent for this movement and the foot can be performed in a wrapped or basic *cou-de-pied*. The standing foot can be flat on the ground (*à terre*) or on demi-pointe (sur la *demi-pointe*).

Piqué meaning "pricking." A *piqué* is performed by stepping directly onto pointe or *demi-pointe* of the standing leg with a straight knee. The working knee is bent, with the working toe placed by the standing knee. The term *piqué* describes how a dancer transfers weight onto the leg going on pointe and can be used in conjunction with other positions like piqué *arabesque* and piqué *passé*.

Plié meaning "bent" or "bending." A *plié* is a bending of the knees, usually performed in one of the six positions of the feet: first, second, third, fourth, fifth, or sixth. *Demi-plié* is a small, or half bend of the knees, keeping the heels of the feet flat on the floor. *Grand plié* is a full or large bend of the knees. In a *grand plié* the legs bend deeply enough so that the heels come off the floor at the bottom of the *plié* in all positions except second.

Sauté meaning "jump." Every jump is technically a *sauté*. The type depends upon the position of the body in the air. For example, a *sauté arabesque* is a jump in *arabesque*.

Sissonne a jump where a dancer pushes off the floor with two feet, splitting their legs in the air "like scissors" and landing. The landing can be on either one or two feet depending on the type of *sissonne*.

Sous-Sus meaning "over, under." In a *sous-sus* the back foot is placed very close behind the front foot, either in *demi-pointe* or full *pointe*, squeezing the legs together into a tight fifth position while keeping both legs fully straight.

Supporting Leg the supporting, or standing leg, describes the leg bearing weight and supporting the entire body while the other, or "working leg," is free to perform a movement or position.

Tendu meaning "tight" or "stretched." A *tendu* is one of the fundamental movements in ballet where the working leg is extended along the floor until only the tip of the toe remains touching the floor. It can be performed to the front, side, or back and usually begins in first or fifth position. *Tendu* is the common abbreviation for a battement *tendu*, and is often used in preparation for larger movements like *grands* battements.

Working Leg the leg that is executing a given movement or position.

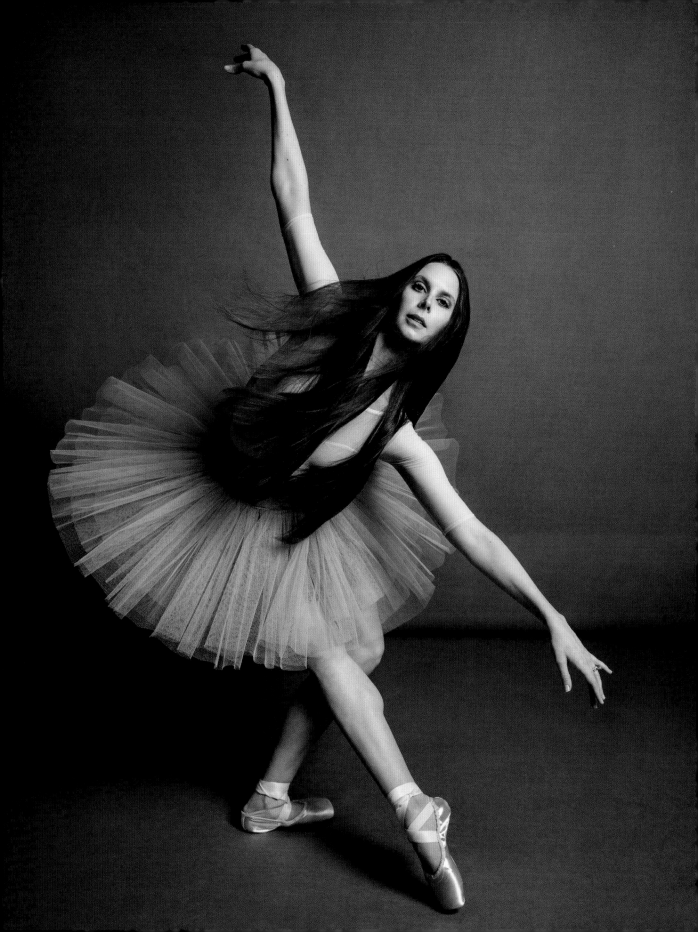

Acknowledgments

Ballet Beautiful is more than a workout; it is an outlook on life. I owe a debt of gratitude to many. My deepest thanks to all the friends, family, and our many fans around the globe who have helped build this incredible movement and company. I would not be here without all of you!

Working with Rizzoli is a dream come true. To Charles, my wonderful editor Caitlin, and the entire Rizzoli team—thank you for your vision and guidance in bringing this very special book to life.

To Inez and Vinoodh, a huge hug and endless thanks to both of you for bringing so much beauty to this world! I will forever treasure working with you on this project. You capture the essence of Ballet Beautiful. Thank you for the marvelous photographs. Many thanks, too, for leading me to the fabulous Chris Colls. Chris, your photos are one of a kind. Thank you for the beautiful images. Harry, thank you for making our Ballet Beautiful meals picture perfect. Peter, you brought it all together on the page in the most magical way. To Jeanine, your friendship and support means so much. Thanks to Aki, Deborah, and Kumiko for making me my most beautiful on camera.

To our amazing Ballet Beauties, thank you for making Ballet Beautiful a part of your daily life, for your sunshine, and your support. To Lily, working out with you never feels like work! Thank you for sharing your Ballet Beautiful story with us all, and for your incredible dedication and mommy advice. You put the "super" in super mama! Alexa, Doutzen, Natalie, Raquel, Liv, Imaan, Gigi, Miranda, Dree, Carolyn, Kristina, Lauren, Karen, Vanessa, Erin, Haley, Phoebe, Stephanie, Jaimie, Carine, Julia, Ray, Tara, Dakota, Christina, Ray, Karlie, Yelena, Anne, and so many others, thank you for the friendship, inspiration, and love.

To the incredible Ballet Beautiful team, thank you for making Ballet Beautiful all that it is and for giving us the ability to strengthen and empower so many. Eliza, your unique eye and attention to detail helps set the stage for all we do. Thank you for your boundless positive energy and many contributions that made this project truly Ballet Beautiful. Max, you bring our vision to life on screen, helping us to share Ballet Beautiful with the world. Nicole and Anna, your support makes every day so smooth. Yuki, Samantha, Nicholas, and our amazing master trainers who help us share the workout with New York City and beyond, thank you for your hard work, sweat, and dedication.

And finally, to my family, who inspires me everyday. Thank you for the love and endless laughs! To Paul, for fifteen years of unwavering support, two beautiful daughters, a thousand cups of coffee, hugs, and homemade meals, thank you. To Lumina and Violette, being your mother is the greatest gift of my life. And to my Mom and Dad, we would not have made it without your babysitting, homemade biscuits, and all-around support. Thank you for teaching me the value of hard work, dedication, and that no dream is ever out of reach.

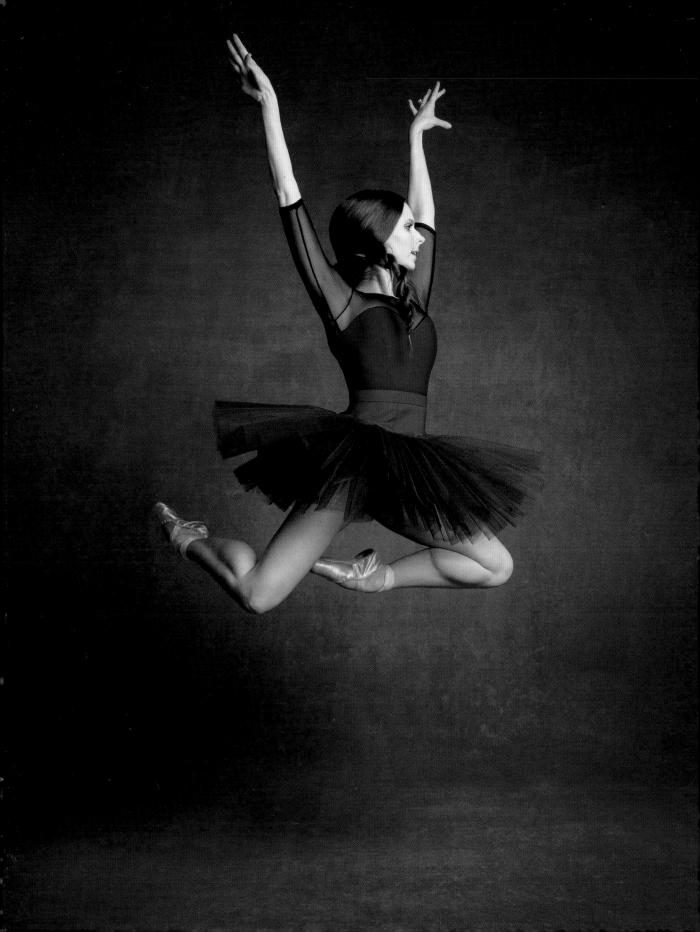

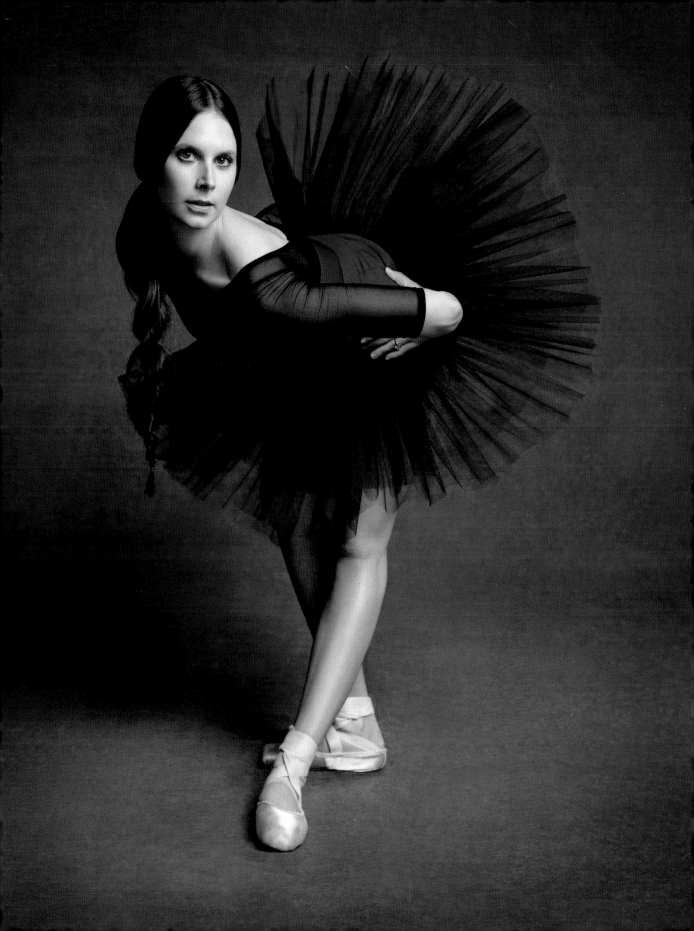

First published in the United States of America
in 2017 by:

Rizzoli International Publications, Inc.
300 Park Avenue South
New York, NY 10010
www.rizzoliusa.com

ISBN: 9780847858378
Library of Congress Control Number: 2016956273

Distributed to the US Trade by
Random House, New York

Design & Custom Lettering:
AHL&CO / Peter J. Ahlberg, Alex Stikeleather

Photography by Inez and Vinoodh: Pages 1, 4, 6, 7, 8,
9, 10, 11, 12-13, 14, 17, 18, 28, 46, 66, 84, 104, 122-3,
148, 152-3, 154, 155, 156-7, 160, 163, 190, 191.

Photography by Chris Colls: 31, 32, 33, 34, 35, 38, 39,
40, 41, 42-3, 44, 45, 49, 50, 51, 52, 53, 54-5, 57, 58, 59,
60, 61, 62, 63, 64, 65, 69, 70, 71, 73, 74-5, 76, 77, 78-9,
80, 81, 82, 83, 87, 88-9, 90-1, 92-3, 94-5, 96, 97, 98, 99,
101, 102-3, 107, 108-9, 116, 117, 118, 119, 120-1, 125,
126-7, 128, 129, 130, 131, 132-3, 134-5, 136-7, 138-9,
140-1, 142-3, 151, 158, 159, 166-7, 168, 169, 170-1.

Photography by Harry Zernike: 172, 175, 176, 177,
178-9, 180, 181, 182, 183, 184-5.

Photography by Ballet Beautiful: 164-5.

All dance clothes, slippers, leotards, tutus, tights, and
tops by Ballet Beautiful.

2017 2018 2019 2020 / 10 9 8 7 6 5 4 3 2 1

Printed in China